Workbook for

Radiographic Image Analysis

Workbook for

Radiographic Image Analysis

Sixth Edition

Kathy McQuillen Martensen, MA, RT(R)
Associate of Radiology
Roy J. and Lucille A. Carver College of Medicine
University of Iowa
Iowa City, Iowa

Stephanie Harris, BS, RT(R)(M)(CT)
Director, Hospital Ambulatory Services
Mercy Hospital
Cedar Rapids, Iowa

ELSEVIER

Elsevier
3251 Riverport Lane
St. Louis, Missouri 63043

WORKBOOK FOR RADIOGRAPHIC IMAGE ANALYSIS,
SIXTH EDITION

ISBN: 978-0-323-93068-0

Previous editions copyrighted 2020, 2015, 2011, 2006, and 1996.

Content Strategist: Meg Benson
Senior Content Development Specialist: Vaishali Singh
Publishing Services Manager: Deepthi Unni
Project Manager: Sindhuraj Thulasingam
Design Direction: Gopalakrishnan Venkatraman

Printed in India

Last digit is the print number: 9 8 7 6 5 4 3 2 1

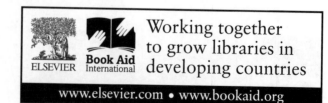

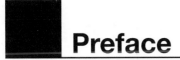

Preface

This workbook has been designed to provide students with a means of testing their understanding of the information covered in the *Radiographic Image Analysis* textbook. It follows the same format as the textbook, with the first two chapters focusing on the image analysis guidelines, and technical and digital imaging concepts that are considered when all procedures are evaluated for quality. The workbook includes questions and projections to evaluate for each of the image analysis guidelines, and technical and digital concepts presented in the first two chapters of *Radiographic Image Analysis*. The remaining chapters guide the student through the image analysis procedural process of each body structure in a systematic fashion. The chapters can be followed as written, or the student may skip from chapter to chapter or procedure to procedure.

For these chapters, the workbook provides the following features for each procedure presented:

■ Study questions that focus on how the patient should be positioned to obtain an accurately positioned projection and what guidelines should be present when proper positioning is obtained. Also, some questions concentrate on improperly positioned projections. The student is asked to state how the patient, CR, or IR was mispositioned to obtain such a projection.

■ Poorly positioned projections that separately focus on each topic and procedure. The projections are different from those found in the textbook and sometimes present multiple positioning problems. Nonroutine scenarios are also presented.

■ Answer keys to the study questions are found on the Evolve Resources for *Radiographic Image Analysis*.

STUDENT GUIDELINES

Prerequisite: It is suggested that a course in anatomy and basic medical terminology be taken before studying radiographic procedures and analysis. For best understanding, it is effective to study the radiographic procedure in conjunction with the analysis.

Guideline 1: Read the learning objectives provided in the *Radiographic Image Analysis* textbook for the chapter being studied. These objectives outline key issues within the chapter and identify the knowledge you should understand after the chapter has been studied.

Guideline 2: Read the corresponding chapter in *Radiographic Image Analysis* and attend the procedure and analysis courses that focus on the subject matter.

Guideline 3: Fill in as many of the study question blanks as you can without referring to the textbook or the workbook answer key. Any blanks that you were unable to complete indicate the areas that require further study. If you left any questions unanswered or if you were uncertain of the correct answers, restudy the information covered in those questions.

Guideline 4: Check your study question answers with the answers provided in the Evolve Resources. Restudy the information covered in any questions you answered incorrectly.

Guideline 5: Consult with your instructor about taking a final examination.

Contents

1 Guidelines for Image Analysis

STUDY QUESTIONS

1. An optimal radiographic projection demonstrates what desired features?

   A. _____

   B. _____

   C. _____

   D. _____

   E. _____

   F. _____

   G. _____

   H. _____

   I. _____

   J. _____

Using the Key Terms listed at the beginning of Chapter 1 in the *Radiographic Image Analysis* textbook, complete the following.

2. Use the lateral chest drawing in Figure 1-1 to complete the following statements.

Figure 1-1

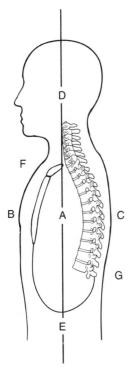

   A. Letter A is situated on the _____ plane.

   B. Letter B is placed _____ to letter A.

   C. Letter C is placed _____ to letter A.

   D. Letter D is placed _____ to letter A.

   E. Letter E is placed _____ to letter A.

   F. Letter F is placed _____ to letter A.

   G. Letter G is placed _____ to letter A.

3. The inferior scapular angle moves toward the front and outer edge of the body when the humerus is abducted. What combination of the positioning terms is used to describe this movement? _____

4. When the humerus is brought from an abducted position to the patient's side, the inferior scapular angle moves toward the patient's back and closer to the midsagittal plane. What combination of the positioning terms is used to describe this movement? _____

5. What combination of the positioning terms is used to describe the portion of the scapula that is positioned closest to the patient's front and head? _____

6. If the IR was placed against the lateral aspect of the leg for a lateral lower leg projection and the CR was centered to the medial aspect, what projection of the leg was taken? _____

7. Use the abdominal drawing in Figure 1-2 to complete the following statements.

Figure 1-2

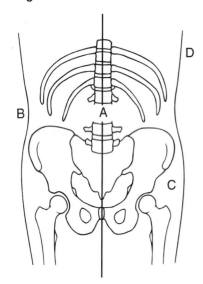

A. Letter A is situated on the _____ plane.

B. Letter B is placed _____ to letter A.

C. Letter A is placed _____ to letter B.

D. Letter C is placed _____ to letter A.

E. Letter D is placed _____ to letter A.

8. Use the drawing of the knee in Figure 1-3 to complete the following statements.

Figure 1-3

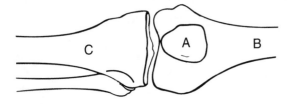

A. Letter B is placed _____ to letter A.

B. Letter C is placed _____ to letter A.

9. State the distances indicated in Figure 1-4.

Figure 1-4

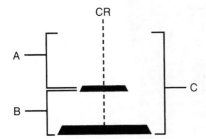

A. _____

B. _____

C. _____

10. Use the following (1 to 6) to define how radiographic projections of the listed body parts are accurately displayed on the monitor.
    1. Displayed as if the patient were standing upright
    2. Displayed as if hanging from the fingertips
    3. Displayed as if hanging from the shoulders
    4. Displayed as if hanging from the toes
    5. Displayed as if hanging from the hip
    6. Displayed as if hanging from the anterior surface

    A. _____ Chest

    B. _____ Wrist

    C. _____ Lumbar vertebrae

    D. _____ Humerus

    E. _____ Toes

    F. _____ Oblique foot

    G. _____ Lateral foot

    H. _____ Ankle

    I. _____ Lower leg

    J. _____ AP hip

    K. _____ Axiolateral shoulder

    L. _____ Cervical vertebrae

    M. _____ Abdomen

11. Evaluate the following projections for displaying accuracy.

Figure 1-5

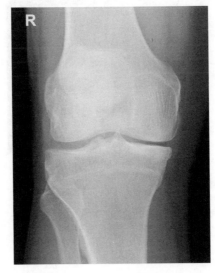

A. AP knee (Figure 1-5): _____

_____

Figure 1-6

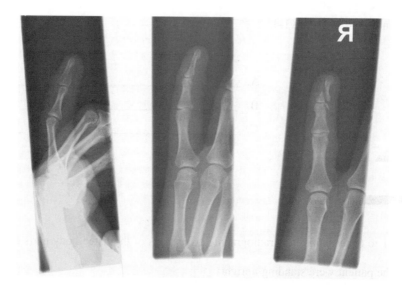

B. Right finger (Figure 1-6): _____

_____

Figure 1-7

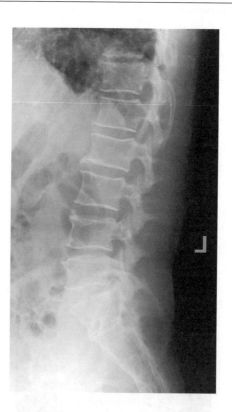

C. Left lateral lumbar vertebrae (Figure 1-7): _____

_____

Figure 1-8

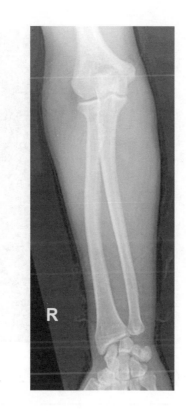

D. AP right forearm (Figure 1-8): _____

_____

Figure 1-9

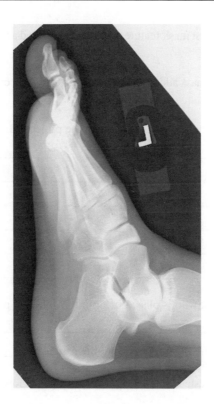

E. Mediolateral left foot (Figure 1-9): _____

_____

5

Figure 1-10

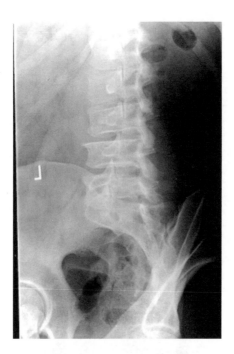

F. AP oblique (LPO) lumbar vertebrae (Figure 1-10): _____

_____

12. When an AP/PA projection or AP/PA oblique projection of the torso is accurately displayed, the patient's right side is on the viewer's _____ side.

13. When using the postprocessing contrast mask feature, only the unexposed areas are masked. _____ (True/False)

14. A projection that has had the contrast mask added and was saved to the PACS can be unmasked. _____ (True/False)

15. List the demographic information that is to be displayed on the projection.

A. _____

B. _____

C. _____

D. _____

E. _____

F. _____

16. A. What marker is used for a patient who is placed in a right PA oblique projection (RAO position)?

_____

B. Where is the marker placed on the IR in reference to the patient? _____

17. A lateral vertebral projection is requested, and the right side is placed closest to the IR.

A. What marker is used for a patient in this projection? _____

B. Where is the marker placed on the IR in reference to the patient? _____

18. Evaluate the following projections for marker placement accuracy.

Figure 1-11

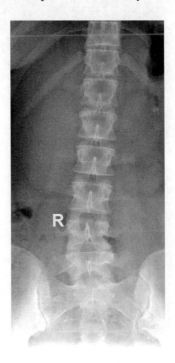

A. AP lumbar vertebrae (Figure 1-11): _____

_____

Figure 1-12

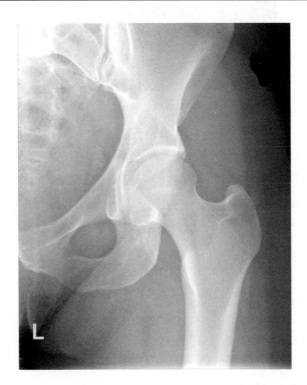

B. AP left hip (Figure 1-12): _____

_____

Chapter **1 Guidelines for Image Analysis**

Figure 1-13

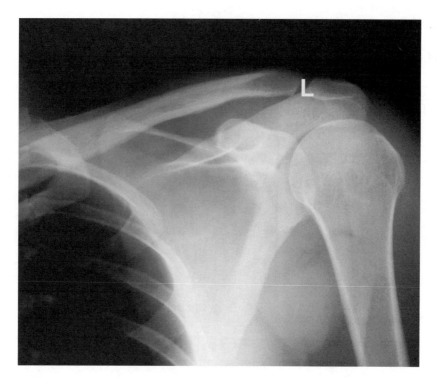

C. AP left shoulder (Figure 1-13): _____

_____

Figure 1-14

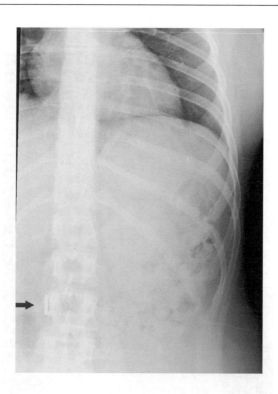

D. AP left lower ribs (Figure 1-14): _____

_____

Figure 1-15

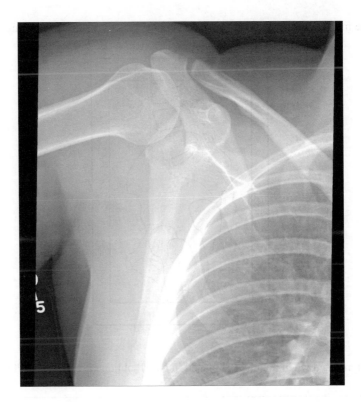

E. AP right scapula (Figure 1-15): _____

_____

19. The markers used in radiography are constructed of (A) _____ and are (B) _____ (radiolucent/radiopaque).

20. The marker placed on a lateral projection of the torso or skull represents the side of the patient that is positioned _____ (closer to/farther from) the IR.

21. Place an R where the marker should be positioned on the hip diagram in Figure 1-16.

Figure 1-16

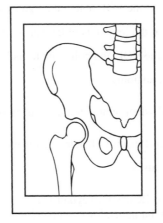

Chapter **1 Guidelines for Image Analysis**

22. Place an L where the marker should be positioned on the lateral sacral diagram in Figure 1-17.

Figure 1-17

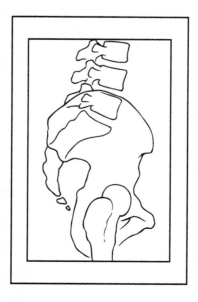

23. How is the projection marked when a patient is placed in an AP oblique projection (LPO or RPO position)?

_____

_____

24. What procedure is followed when the marker has not been demonstrated within the exposure field but is only faintly seen along its border?

_____

25. Good collimation practices clearly delineate the VOI, (A) _____ (increase/decrease) patient radiation dosage, (B) _____ (increase/decrease) the visibility of recorded details, and (C) _____ (increase/decrease) histogram analysis errors.

26. To provide even collimation on all sides of the VOI, obtain the tightest collimation and provide the best positioning for good exposure field recognition, align the long axis of the part to the (A) _____ of the IR, center the (B) _____ to the center of the VOI, and collimate to include only the VOI and (C) _____ _____ of the surrounding anatomy.

27. The display screen is filled with the VOI when tight collimation is used. _____ (True/False)

28. The tube column can be rotated for a grid exam to better align it with an anatomical structure and obtain tighter collimation. _____ (True/False)

29. Describe why it is necessary to have the IR extend beyond the joint spaces by 1 to 2 inches (2.5 to 5 cm) when imaging long bones such as the forearm, humerus, lower leg, and femur.

_____

_____

Figure 1-18

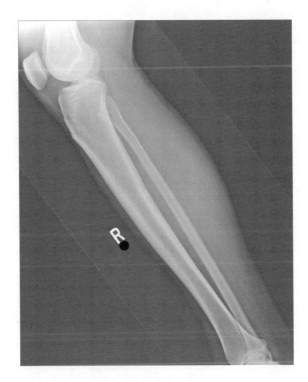

30. Evaluate the accuracy of the placement of the anatomic structures on the IR in Figure 1-18.

_____

_____

Figure 1-19

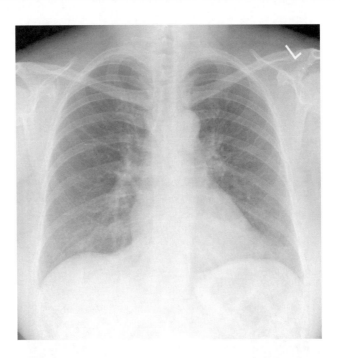

31. State where the CR was centered on the projection in Figure 1-19.

_____

32. The collimator's light field that is demonstrated on the patient's abdomen in Figure 1-20 measures 8 × 10 inches (18 × 24 cm). Does this mean that the IR exposure field coverage will be 8 × 10 inches, or should it be larger or smaller?

Figure 1-20

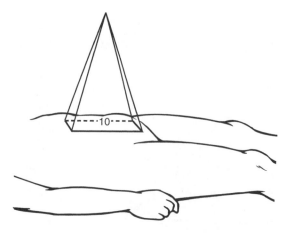

A. _____

Explain your answer.

B. _____

33. Contrast masking is an acceptable postprocessing manipulation that can be used to reduce the amount of anatomical

structures seen on the projection. _____ (True/False)

34. Evaluate the following projections for good collimation practices and state how poor CR centering has prevented tighter collimation.

Figure 1-21

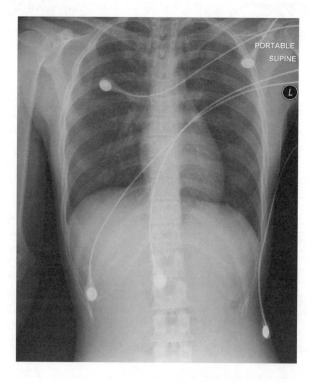

A. Figure 1-21 AP chest _____

Figure 1-22

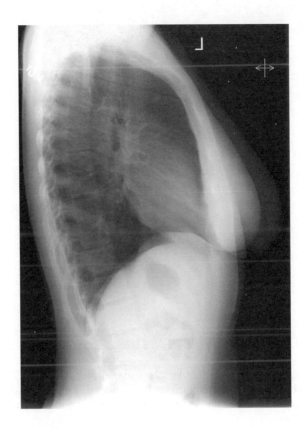

B. Figure 1-22 Lateral chest _____

Figure 1-23

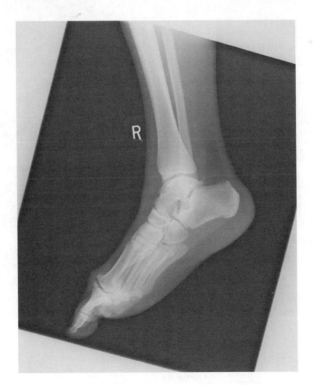

C. Figure 1-23 Lateral foot _____

Figure 1-24

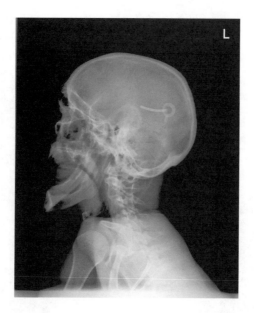

D. Figure 1-24 Lateral skull _____

35. Tighter collimation was obtained on one of the AP clavicular projections in Figure 1-25 with the tube column rotated, and the other was obtained with the collimator head rotated. Indicate below the clavicular projection that was obtained with the tube column rotated and the projection obtained with the collimator head rotated.

Figure 1-25

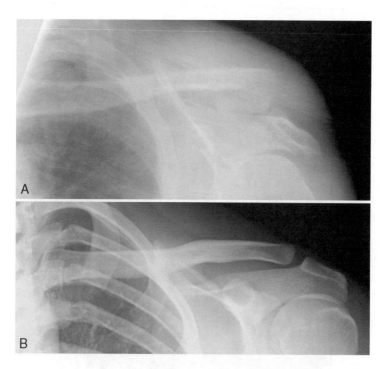

A. Tube column rotation: _____ (A or B)

B. Collimator head rotation: _____ (A or B)

C. Defend your answers to A and B above. _____

_____

36. Use the lateral knee diagram in Figure 1-26 to answer the following questions.

Figure 1-26

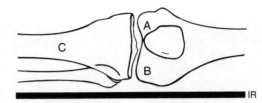

IR

A. If a perpendicular CR was centered to letter A on the knee diagram, where would letter A be positioned in reference to letter B on the resulting radiographic projection?

_____

B. If a perpendicular CR was centered to the letter C on the knee diagram, where would letter A be positioned in reference to letter B on the resulting projection?

(1) _____

Will both letter A and letter B be projected the same distance?

(2) _____ (Yes/No)

Defend your answer.

(3) _____

C. If the CR was angled 15 degrees caudally and centered to letter A on the knee diagram, where would letter A be positioned in reference to letter B on the projection?

(1) _____

How would the projection change if the CR angulation was increased to 45 degrees?

(2) _____

D. If the CR was angled 15 degrees caudally and centered to letter C on the knee diagram, where would letter A be positioned in reference to letter B on the projection?

_____

_____

37. Eight soup cans were arranged on top of a 14 × 17-inch IR as shown in Figures 1-27 and 1-28. A perpendicular CR was centered to the center of the IR. The circles that are demonstrated indicate the bottom of each soup can that is 4 inches (10 cm) tall. Draw a second circle for each of the cans to indicate where the top of the soup can will be located on the resulting projection. You must consider the direction the top of the can will be projected because of diverged beams that will be used to record them and the degree of off-centering from the bottom of the can that will be demonstrated when compared with the other cans.

Figure 1-27

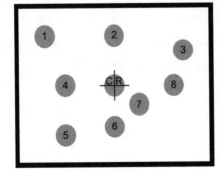

Figure 1-28

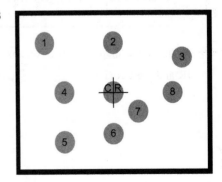

A. On Figure 1-27, draw the circles for an SID of 72 inches (180 cm).
B. On Figure 1-28, draw the circles for an SID of 40 inches (100 cm).

15

38. The AP chest projection in Figure 1-29 was taken using a 48-inch SID and a perpendicular CR. With this as your reference point, answer the following.

Figure 1-29

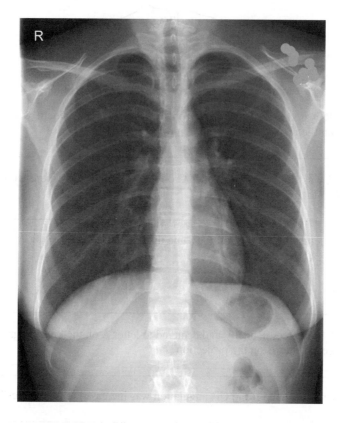

A. If the CR was inadvertently angled 10 degrees toward the right side of the patient, where would the sternoclavicular joints be located in reference to the vertebral column on the resulting AP chest projection?

_____

B. If the CR was angled 10 degrees cephalically, where would the sternoclavicular joints be located in reference to the third thoracic vertebral body?

_____

C. How would your answers to A and B be different if a 72-inch SID were used?

_____

D. How would your answers to A and B be different if the heart shadow was used as your reference point instead of the sternoclavicular joints?

_____

39. To minimize shape distortion on a projection, keep the part positioned (A) _____ (parallel/perpendicular) to the IR and the CR (B) _____ (parallel/perpendicular) to both the part and the IR.

40. For the CR, part, and IR setups in the following figures, state the type of shape distortion that will result.

Figure 1-30

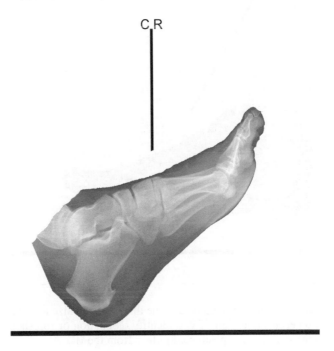

A. Figure 1-30 _____

Figure 1-31

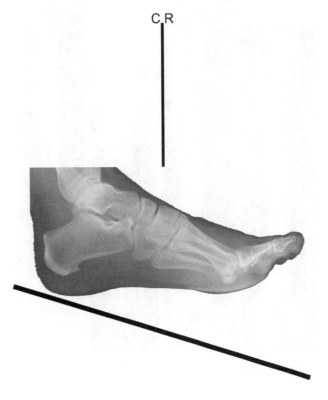

B. Figure 1-31 _____

Figure 1-32

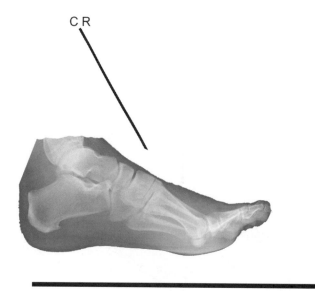

C R

C. Figure 1-32 _____

41. Figure 1-33 demonstrates AP projections of a humeral bone that has been size and shape distorted. Identify the type of distortion demonstrated on each projection. If you identify elongation or foreshortening, state the aspect of the bone (proximal or distal humerus) that was positioned farther from the IR.

Figure 1-33

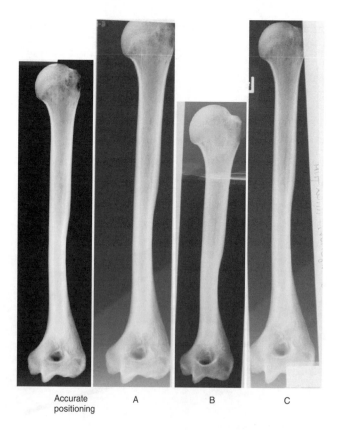

Accurate positioning   A   B   C

A. _____

B. _____

C. _____

42. Which of the following images will have the greater part magnification?
Image 1 was exposed at a 72-inch SID and a 3-inch OID.
Image 2 was exposed at a 72-inch SID and a 4-inch OID.

43. Which of the following images will have the greater part magnification?
Image 1 was exposed at a 72-inch SID and a 2-inch OID.
Image 2 was exposed at a 40-inch SID and a 2-inch OID.

44. List three ways of identifying similarly appearing structures from one another on a projection.

A. _____

B. _____

C. _____

45. If two structures are demonstrated without superimposition on a mispositioned projection and they should be superimposed on an accurately positioned image of this projection, how does one determine how much to adjust the patient to obtain an optimal projection if both structures move in opposite directions when adjusted?

A. _____

If only one structure moved when the patient was adjusted?

B. _____

46. Estimate the degree of patient obliquity demonstrated in the diagrams in Figure 1-34.

Figure 1-34

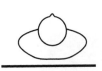

A. _____ degrees

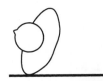

B. _____ degrees

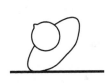

C. _____ degrees

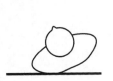

D. _____ degrees

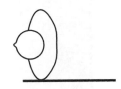

E. _____ degrees

47. Estimate the degree of flexion demonstrated in the following figures.

Figure 1-35

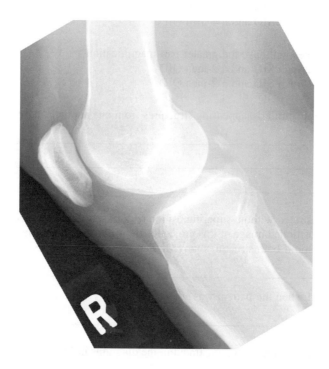

A. _____ degrees (Figure 1-35)

Figure 1-36

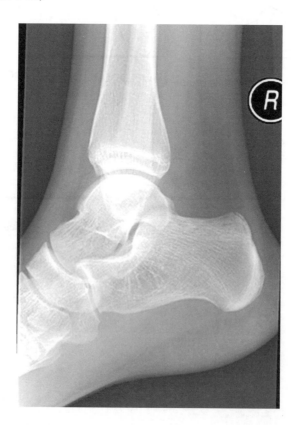

B. _____ degrees (Figure 1-36)

Figure 1-37

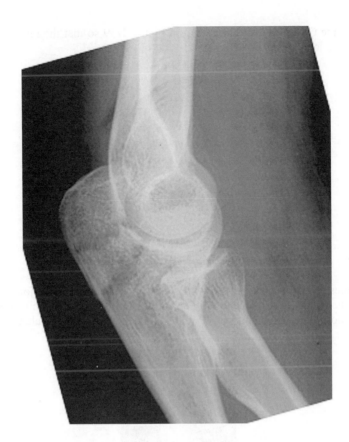

C. _____ degrees (Figure 1-37)

Figure 1-38

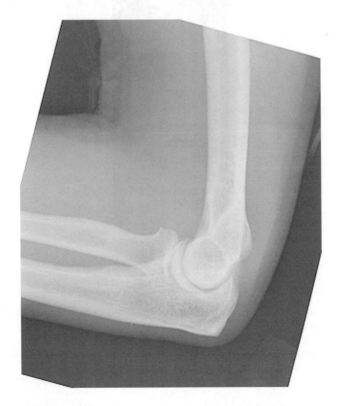

D. _____ degrees (Figure 1-38)

48. Draw a line to indicate the CR on the AP knee setup in Figure 1-39 so that the resulting AP knee projection will demonstrate an open knee joint space.

Figure 1-39

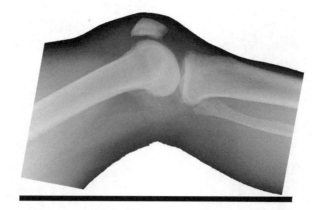

49. Figure 1-40 demonstrates a PA finger projection with closed interphalangeal (IP) joints and foreshortened middle and distal phalanges. The patient was unable to fully extend the finger for the examination. Explain how the central ray and part should be positioned to obtain open IP joints and demonstrate the phalanges without foreshortening.

Figure 1-40

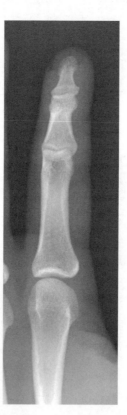

A. _____

Explain how the technologist would have to adjust the CR to obtain open IP joints and nonforeshortened phalanges if the patient were unable to adjust the hand.

B. _____

_____

50. An angled CR projects the structure situated (A) _____ (closer to/farther from) the IR farther than a structure situated (B) _____ (closer to/farther from) the IR.

22

51. Figure 1-41 demonstrates an accurately and poorly positioned lateral hand projection. On the poorly positioned projection, the fifth metacarpal (MC) is situated 1 inch (2.5 cm) anterior to the second through fourth MCs. The second through fifth MCs should be superimposed on an optimal lateral hand projection. The physical distance between the second and fifth MCs is 2½ inches (6.25 cm).

Figure 1-41

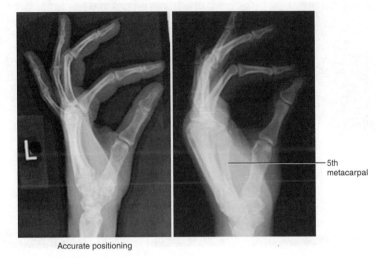

Accurate positioning

5th metacarpal

A. State how and by how much the patient's positioning should be adjusted to obtain an optimal projection. The second and fifth MCs will move in opposite directions from each other when the hand is rotated.

_____

B. State how the CR could be directed toward the hand and the amount of angulation needed to obtain an optimal projection if the patient were unable to adjust positioning.

_____

52. Figure 1-42 demonstrates an accurately and a poorly positioned lateral knee projection. On the poorly positioned projection, the lateral femoral condyle is situated 2 inches (5 cm) anterior to the medial femoral condyle. The condyles should be superimposed on an optimal lateral knee projection. The physical distance between the femoral condyles is 2½ inches (6.25 cm).

Figure 1-42

Medial condyle

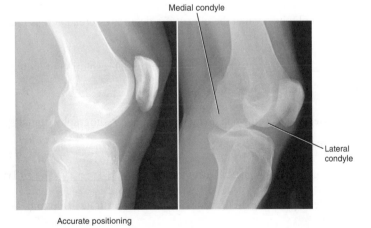

Lateral condyle

Accurate positioning

A. State how and by how much the patient's positioning could be adjusted to obtain an optimal projection. The lateral and medial condyles will move in opposite directions from each other when the knee is rotated.

_____

B. State how the CR should be directed toward the knee and the amount of angulation needed to obtain an optimal projection if the patient were unable to adjust positioning.

_____

_____

53. Figure 1-43 demonstrates an accurately and a poorly positioned lateral ankle projection. On the poorly positioned projection, the lateral talar dome is situated ¼ inch (0.6 cm) posterior to the medial dome. The talar domes should be superimposed on an optimal lateral ankle projection. The physical distance between the talar domes is 1 inch (2.5 cm).

Figure 1-43

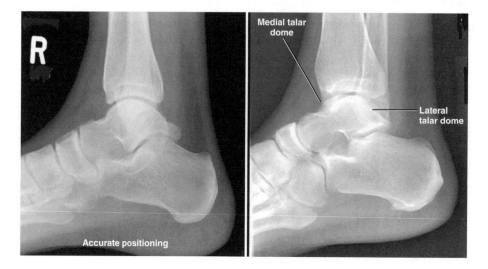

A. State how and by how much the patient's positioning could be adjusted to obtain an optimal projection. The lateral and medial talar domes will move in opposite directions from each other when the ankle is rotated.

_____

B. State how the CR should be directed toward the ankle and the amount of angulation needed to obtain an optimal projection if the patient were unable to adjust positioning.

_____

54. Spatial resolution refers to the ability of the imaging system to record sharp detail edges and distinguish small adjacent details from each other in a projection. _____ (True/False)

55. Sharpness of a detail has been obtained when the edges of a detail are spread across many pixels. _____ (True/False)

56. The term (A) _____ is used to describe the spatial resolution of a digital system and refers to the number of details that can be visualized in a set (B) _____.

57. The smallest possible IR cassette is chosen when using the computer radiography digital system to produce a projection with maximum spatial resolution. _____ (True/False)

58. DR system's pixel sizes change with a change in collimation. _____ (True/False)

59. DR system A can demonstrate 5 lp/mm, and DR system B can demonstrate 10 lp/mm. Which system demonstrates the greatest spatial resolution?

_____

60. An AP pelvis and an AP hip projection were obtained using the same computed radiography system. State which projection will demonstrate the greatest spatial resolution and explain why.

_____

61. When obtaining a projection using a DR system, greater spatial resolution is obtained when the technologist collimates to a smaller area. _____ (True/False)

24

62. A _____ (large/small) focal spot size is used for fine detail demonstration because a detail that is _____ (larger/smaller) than the focal spot size used to produce the projection will not be demonstrated.

63. A _____ (longer/shorter) SID and a _____ (longer/shorter) OID will produce the sharpest recorded details on a projection.

64. List four ways that voluntary motion can be controlled.

   A. _____

   B. _____

   C. _____

   D. _____

65. How can voluntary and involuntary motion be distinguished from each other on a supine abdominal projection?

   _____

   _____

66. State whether the following situations are examples of voluntary or involuntary motions.

   A. The patient was extremely short of breath because of asthma and unable to hold it.

   _____

   B. After being in a car accident, the patient being imaged was unable to stop shaking.

   _____

67. The projection in Figure 1-44 demonstrates poor radiation protection practices. What type of error is demonstrated?

   A. _____

   How could this examination be taken without this error?

   B. _____

Figure 1-44

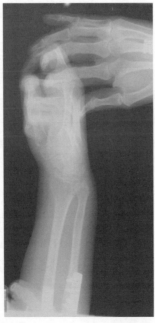

68. The technologist sets up for a routine AP abdomen projection on an obese patient using the mobile radiography unit. The resulting SSD is 10 inches (25 cm). Using appropriate radiation protection practices, state how the setup should be adjusted before exposing the projection. _____

25

2 Visibility of Details

1. The peaks and valleys in the histogram represent the (A) _____ in the remnant radiation and is determined by the total (B) _____ that is used to create the latent image.

2. On a histogram graph, what is identified on the following?

   A. x-axis: _____

   B. y-axis: _____

3. The VOI on a histogram graph identifies S_{min} as the _____ (minimal/maximal) gray shade value.

4. Rank the following in the order each is demonstrated on a histogram, with 1 being farthest to the left on the graph and 5 being farthest to the right.

   _____ Air/gas

   _____ Bone

   _____ Contrast/metal

   _____ Fat

   _____ Soft tissue

5. The _____ represents the ideal histogram for the projection.

6. During the exposure field recognition process, how does the computer identify the VOI?

   _____

7. Describe the three types of histogram analysis that are applied to image histograms.

   A. _____

   B. _____

   C. _____

8. If the VOI on the image histogram were positioned farther to the left than on the LUT, how would the displayed projection appear if rescaling didn't take place?

   _____

9. If the VOI on the image histogram were wider than on the LUT, how would the displayed projection appear if rescaling didn't take place?

   _____

10. Where does the EI reading come from?

_____

11. The ideal EI indicates the (A) _____ gray value and usually represents the

(B) _____.

12. Why do histogram analysis errors produce poor-quality projections?

_____

13. What are the common causes of poor histogram formation (histogram analysis errors)?

A. _____

B. _____

C. _____

D. _____

E. _____

F. Computed radiography only: _____

G. Computed radiography only: _____

H. Computed radiography only: _____

14. In computed radiography, histogram analysis errors can occur because of the projection being improperly centered to the IR or all collimated borders not shown or aligned accurately. Why does this error <u>not</u> occur in DR imaging?

_____

Figure 2-1

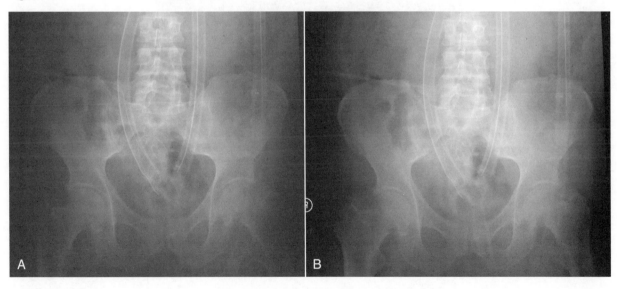

15. Figure 2-1A–B: Determine which AP abdomen projection was processed under a chest LUT and which was processed under an abdomen LUT. (Hint: Look at the contrast of each projection.)

_____

_____

_____

16. How can the reviewer know that a projection was processed under an alternate algorithm?

_____

Figure 2-2 Lateral lumbar spine

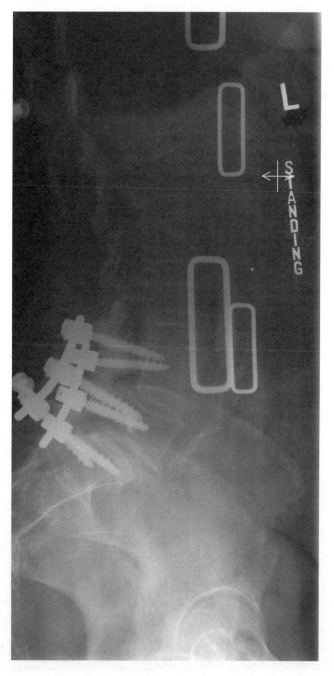

17. Describe the histogram analysis error that is demonstrated and why it occurred in Figure 2-2.

_____

Figure 2-3 Upright AP abdomen

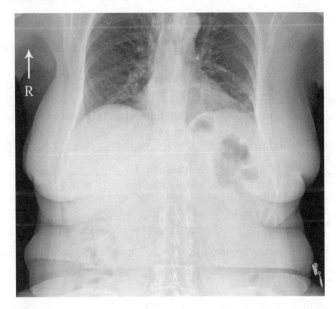

18. Describe the histogram analysis error that is demonstrated and why it occurred in Figure 2-3. _____

_____

19. The degree of contrast resolution present on projections is determined by the:

A. _____

B. _____

C. _____

20. Indicate whether projections on patients with the following will display high (H) or low (L) subject contrast.

_____ A. Strong muscles

_____ B. Dense bones

_____ C. Fluid retention caused by disease or injury

_____ D. Porous bones

_____ E. High fat

_____ F. Bones of infants

_____ G. Obesity

21. List the technical factors that affect the amount of exposure the IR receives.

A. _____

B. _____

C. _____

D. _____

E. _____

F. _____

22. Absorption (PE affect) no longer takes place in (A) _____ when the kVp is set above 80 and will no longer happen in (B) _____ when set above 120 kVp.

23. How does the technologist determine if the bony structures have been adequately penetrated? _____
_____

24. A portion of the VOI that is demonstrated as a pitch-black shade is defined as being _____
as a result of overwhelming the digital system with electronic signals because of extreme exposure.

25. Scatter radiation reaching the IR increases with (A) _____ (thicker/thinner) body parts,
(B) _____ (larger/smaller) field sizes, and (C) _____ (lower/higher) kVp levels.

26. What type of noise results when the exposure reaching the IR is so low that the random distribution of photons on the projection is demonstrated? _____

27. When there is an increase in scatter or quantum noise demonstrated on the projection, the SNR is higher.
_____ (True/False)

28. A high-quality projection will demonstrate the following visibility of detail characteristics.

A. _____
_____

B. _____
_____

C. _____
_____

29. An under- or overexposed projection that is off by a factor of 2 can be rescaled and does not need repeating as long as at least some number of primary x-rays have penetrated through all the tissues. _____ (True/False)

30. An underexposed projection that requires repeating will demonstrate the following characteristics.

A. _____
B. _____
C. _____
D. _____
E. _____

31. List the steps to follow to determine the technical adjustment to make when an underexposed projection is produced.

A. _____
B. _____
C. _____

32. How will the EI be different for an overexposed versus an underexposured projection that does not have to be repeated because it is still within the acceptable exposure parameters? _____

_____

33. An overexposed projection that requires repeating is identified when:

A. _____

B. _____

C. _____

D. _____

E. _____

34. List the subject contrast differences that cause differential absorption and radiographic contrast.

A. _____

B. _____

C. _____

35. What is the technical factor that controls subject contrast and contrast resolution? _____

36. Subject contrast that is not visible on a projection can be recovered with digital postprocessing techniques.

_____ (True/False)

37. Saturation is demonstrated on a projection when details in the VOI demonstrate a(n) (A) _____ shade and occurs when the IR exposure is (B) _____ times more than the ideal.

38. An AP lumbar vertebrae projection was obtained using the Siemens YSIO DR system (EI range 125–500; ideal EI 250), 90 kVp, and 5 mAs. The resulting projection demonstrated adequate penetration of all structures, quantum noise, and a 63 EI number. How should the technical factors be adjusted before repeating the projection?

_____

39. An AP shoulder projection was obtained using the Siemens YSIO DR system (EI range 125–500; ideal EI 250), 80 kVp, and 30 mAs. The resulting projection demonstrated adequate penetration of all structures, no quantum noise, partial saturation of the AC joint and lateral clavicle, and a 750 EI number. What new technical factors should be used for the repeated projection?

_____

40. An AP pelvis projection was obtained using the Carestream CR system, 70 kV, and 5 mAs. The resulting projection demonstrated a lack of subject contrast at the hip joints, quantum noise, and a 1400 EI number. What new technical factors should be used for the repeated projection?

_____

41. How can the amount of scatter radiation reaching the IR be controlled?

A. _____

B. _____

C. _____

Figure 2-4

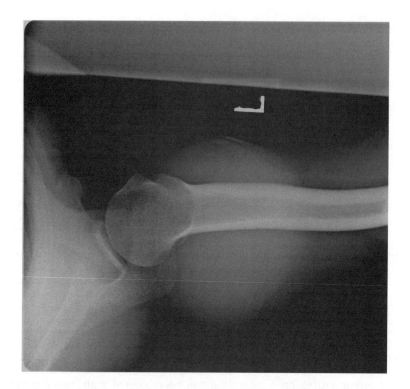

42. Figure 2-4 demonstrates a well-collimated axiolateral (inferosuperior) shoulder projection that demonstrates excessive scatter radiation along the outside of the collimated border. Describe a technique that could be followed to reduce the negative effects of this scatter on the visibility of the recorded details.

_____

43. Use the original technical factors listed below to determine the new mAs that will be needed to produce an optimal projection if the following changes occurred.

Original Technical Factors: 90 kVp, 80 mAs, 8:1 grid

A. Nongrid _____ mAs

B. 6:1 grid _____ mAs

C. 12:1 grid _____ mAs

D. 16:1 grid _____ mAs

44. Indicate whether the following statements are true (T) or false (F) as they relate to grid cutoff.

A. _____ A projection obtained with a tilted focus grid demonstrates grid cutoff on each side.

B. _____ A projection obtained with the focused grid off-centered to the CR demonstrates grid cutoff across the entire projection.

C. _____ A projection obtained with a parallel grid that is inverted demonstrates grid cutoff on each side of the projection.

D. _____ A projection obtained with an off-focused focus grid demonstrates grid cutoff across the entire projection.

45. Grid cutoff resulting from poor grid alignment will be greater on the side the CR is angled (A) _____ (toward/away from), will (B) _____ (increase/decrease) with increased severity of misalignment, and will be more noticeable with (C) _____ (higher/lower) grid ratios.

Figure 2-5 PA chest

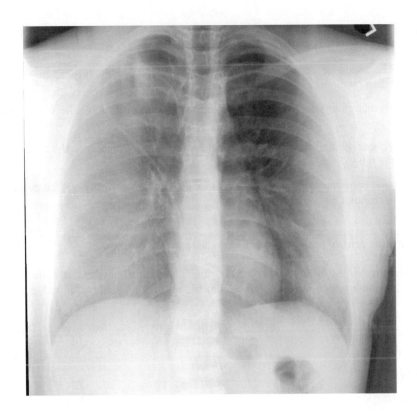

46. State the positioning error that caused the grid alignment artifact that is demonstrated on the PA chest projection in Figure 2-5. _____

47. An optimal AP pelvis projection was obtained in the x-ray department using a 45-inch (113-cm) SID, 80 kVp, and 60 mAs. The next day, the same projection was requested, but because the patient was in traction, the SID needed to be set at a 65-inch (163-cm) SID. What should the new mAs be to obtain an optimal projection?

48. Increasing the OID may result in a significant loss of IR exposure. The amount of loss is dependent on which two factors?

    A. _____

    B. _____

49. When an OID increase causes significant scatter radiation to be diverted from the IR, the technical factor of

    (A) _____ should be increased by (B) _____ percent for every inch of OID increase to compensate for IR exposure loss.

50. State if and by how much the mAs should be adjusted because of increased collimation in the following situations.

    A. PA chest projection was requested to demonstrate the pulmonary arterial catheter. The technologist used 80 kVp at 3 mAs, and the resulting projection did not visualize the catheter tip in the right atrium. To reduce the effects of scatter radiation and demonstrate the catheter tip, the technologist returns to take a second projection, collimating to the VOI (8 × 10 inches). What technique should be used for the second projection?

    _____

    B. Two PA hand projections were obtained on the same patient's hand. A 10- × 12-inch (25- × 30-cm) IR was needed to include the entire hand on the first projection, and the technique used was 60 kVp at 20 mAs. The second projection was collimated to a 2- × 4-inch (5- × 10-cm) field size to include only the first finger. Which technique should be used for the second projection?

    _____

51. Indicate whether the following statements are true (T) or false (F) as they relate to the anode-heel effect by placing a T or F in front of the statement.

_____ A. The anode-heel effect can be used effectively to produce uniform brightness between the toes and foot when obtaining an AP foot projection.

_____ B. To incorporate the anode-heel effect for forearm projections, the wrist is placed at the anode end of the tube.

_____ C. To incorporate the anode-heel effect for lower leg projections, the ankle is placed at the cathode end of the tube.

_____ D. To incorporate the anode-heel effect for an AP thoracic vertebrae, the cephalic end of the patient is placed at the anode end of the tube.

52. A(n) _____ (additive/destructive) type of patient condition causes the tissues to increase mass density or thickness and become more radiopaque.

53. State the technical adjustment needed with the patient condition in the first column and state whether it is an additive or destructive condition, to indicate if the technical adjustment should be increased or decreased by the amount indicated.

	Technical Adjustment	Additive or Destructive
A. Ascites	_____	_____
B. Emphysema	_____	_____
C. Pleural effusion	_____	_____
D. Osteoporosis	_____	_____
E. Osteoarthritis	_____	_____
F. Pneumothorax	_____	_____
G. Pneumonia	_____	_____
H. Bowel obstruction	_____	_____
I. Osteochondroma	_____	_____
J. Rheumatoid arthritis	_____	_____
K. Pulmonary edema	_____	_____
L. Cardiomegaly	_____	_____

54. Indicate whether the following statements are true (T) or false (F) as they relate to proper AEC usage by placing a T or F in front of the statement.

_____ A. Set the kV at optimum for the body part being imaged to obtain appropriate part subject contrast.

_____ B. If the kVp is so low that the part is inadequately penetrated, the exposure (density) control button should be increased to +2.

_____ C. Exposures taken with an exposure time that is less than the minimum response time will result in an overexposed projection.

_____ D. The mA station should be increased if the minimum response time halts the exposure before adequate IR exposure is obtained.

_____ E. The backup time should be set at 150% to 200% of the expected manual exposure time.

_____ F. If the backup time is set at a time that is too low, the exposure will prematurely stop, resulting in an underexposed projection.

_____ G. An overexposed projection results when the ionization chamber chosen is located beneath a structure that has a lower atomic number or is thinner or less dense than the VOI.

_____ H. If the activated ionization chamber is not completely covered by the anatomy, resulting in a portion of the chamber being exposed with a part of the x-ray beam that does not go through the patient, the resulting projection will be underexposed.

_____ I. Scatter radiation may cause the AEC to terminate prematurely.

_____ J. The AEC should not be used when the structure above the ionization chamber varies greatly in thickness.

_____ K. The AEC can be used when radiopaque hardware of prosthetic devices are present as long as the hardware or device is positioned in the center of the chamber.

Figure 2-6 AP hip

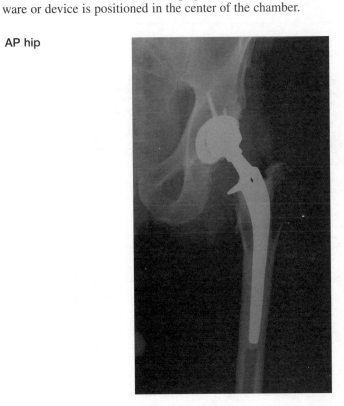

55. Evaluate the following projections for proper AEC usage.

A. AP hip (Figure 2-6) _____

_____ _____

35

Figure 2-7 PA chest

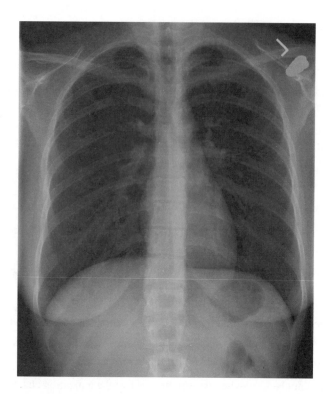

B. PA chest (Figure 2-7) _____

_____

Figure 2-8 Upright AP abdomen, upper projection

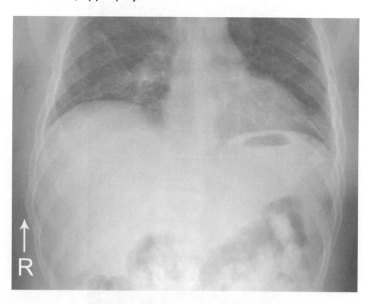

C. Upright AP abdomen, upper projection (Figure 2-8) _____

_____

Figure 2-9 AP shoulder

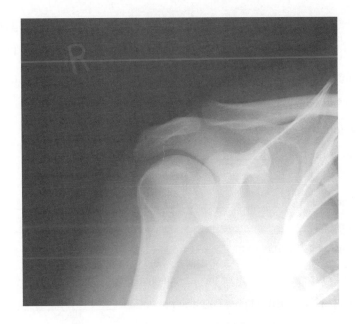

D. AP shoulder (Figure 2-9) _____

_____

Figure 2-10 Lateral lumbar vertebrae

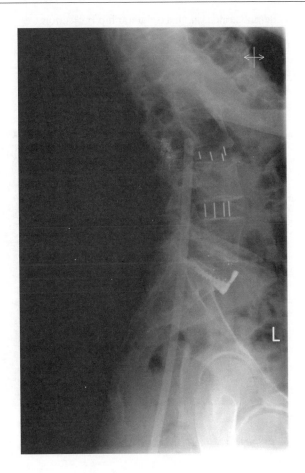

E. Lateral lumbar vertebrae (Figure 2-10) _____

_____

56. Adjusting the window width changes the (A) _____ on the displayed projection, and adjusting the window level changes the (B) _____ of the displayed projection.

57. The technologist should window a less-than-optimal projection and save it to the PACS so the radiologist can display the manipulated projection. _____ (True/False)

58. Describe the following artifact categories.

A. Anatomic artifact: _____

B. Phantom image: _____

C. External artifact: _____

D. Internal artifact: _____

E. Equipment-related artifact: _____

59. State the artifact category for each of the artifacts listed below.

A. A fountain pen is visualized on a PA chest projection. _____

B. A hand is demonstrated on an AP hip projection. _____

C. A prosthesis is demonstrated on an AP shoulder projection. _____

D. Grid cutoff is demonstrated on an axiolateral hip projection. _____

60. Evaluate the following projections for phosphor plate handling artifacts. Choose from the options listed.

1. Dust or dirt   3. Hair

2. Scratches   4. A solution of some type

Figure 2-11

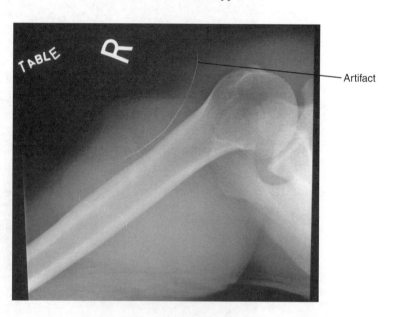

A. _____ Figure 2-11

Figure 2-12

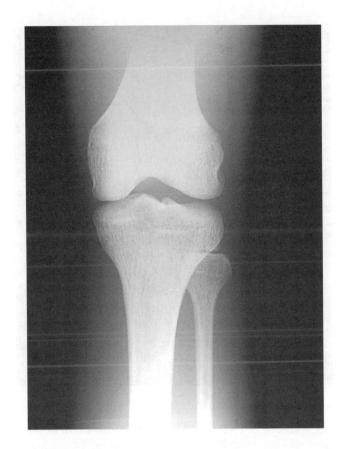

B. _____ Figure 2-12

Figure 2-13

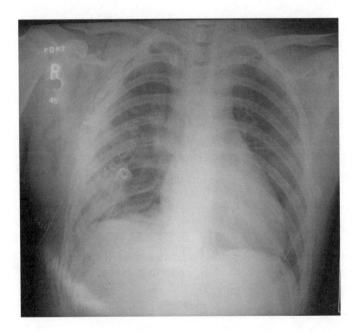

C. _____ Figure 2-13

Figure 2-14

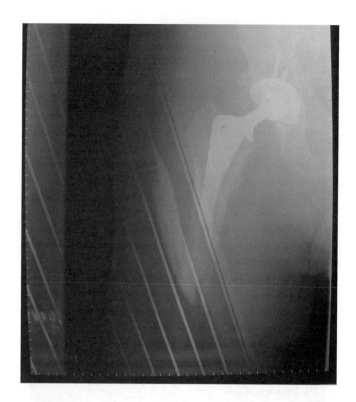

61. Evaluate the mobile AP hip projection in Figure 2-14 to determine the cause of the computed radiography artifact demonstrated. The projection was obtained during morning rounds in the intensive care unit of a busy hospital. Between the ordered examinations, the IR was held in a metal basket until all the projections taken were brought to the department for processing.

_____

62. What is the difference between an optimal and an acceptable projection?

_____

_____

63. When should a projection be repeated because of an artifact?

_____

64. State the goals for performing mobile and trauma imaging.

_____

_____

65. To obtain accurately positioned trauma and mobile projections, the CR-to-part and part-to-IR alignments must be as they routinely are for the projection. For each of the projections below, state the "part" that is aligned with the CR and IR.

A. Lateral hand: _____

B. AP elbow: _____

C. Lateral chest: _____

D. AP oblique (external rotation) knee: _____

E. AP axial cranium (Towne method): _____

40

66. State the technical adjustment needed for trauma patients because of the following.

	kVp Adjustment	mAs Adjustment
A. Small to medium plaster cast	_____	_____
B. Fiberglass cast	_____	_____
C. Wood backboard	_____	_____
D. Postmortem imaging of head, thorax, and abdomen	_____	_____
E. Upper airway obstruction	_____	_____
F. Wood sliver embedded in soft tissue	_____	_____

67. Using the law of isometry, state the degree of CR angulation that is used for the following projections.

    A. If the AP lower leg placed at a 40-degree angle with the IR, place the CR at _____ degrees.

    B. If the AP femur is placed at a 60-degree angle with the IR, place the CR at _____ degrees.

68. A long bone that cannot be positioned with its long axis parallel with the IR will demonstrate the least foreshortening when the law of isometry is used to position the bone and will demonstrate the best anatomic joint relationship when the CR is placed _____ to the bone's long axis.

Figure 2-15

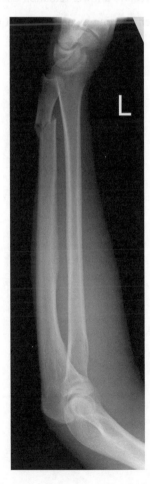

69. The lateral forearm projection in Figure 2-15 demonstrates a distal ulnar fracture. The patient was unable to position the elbow and wrist in a lateral projection at the same time. Evaluate the accuracy of the arm's alignment.

_____

_____

41

70. Indicate whether the following statements are true (T) or false (F) as they relate to pediatric and obese patient imaging by placing a T or F in front of the statement.

_____ A. When imaging pediatric patients, use a high mA and short exposure time to prevent patient motion.

_____ B. Lower the IR exposure by adjusting kV and mAs over those used for adults when imaging pediatric patients to maintain ideal IE exposure.

_____ C. Clothing should be removed when imaging pediatric patients when possible, because the lower kV used increases the chance of clothing artifacts.

_____ D. Using words such as "big" or "lots of help" in hearing distance of an obese patient may make the patient feel unwelcome.

_____ E. Table, wheelchair, and cart weight limits should be determined before using them on an obese patient.

_____ F. Obese patients have inherently high subject contrast.

_____ G. Image contrast is affected by the SNR of scatter-to-primary photons that reach the IR when imaging obese patients.

_____ H. For every 2 cm of added tissue thickness, the mAs should be doubled to maintain IR exposure.

_____ I. If instead of using mAs to maintain IR exposure, the kV was adjusted by 2 for every centimeter of tissue thickness, the patient would receive a lower radiation dose.

_____ J. Using a small focal spot when imaging an obese patient may result in patient motion.

3 Image Analysis of the Chest and Abdomen

STUDY QUESTIONS

1. Complete Figure 3-1.

Figure 3-1

Adult and Pediatric Chest Technical Data					
Projection	kV	Grid	AEC	mAs	SID
Adult Chest Technical Data					
PA					
Lateral					
AP mobile					
AP supine in Bucky					
AP-PA (lateral decubitus)					
AP axial (lordotic)					
Pediatric Chest Technical Data					
Neonate: AP					
Infant: AP					
Child: AP					
Child: PA					
Neonate: Cross-table					
Infant: Cross-table lateral					
Child: Lateral					
Neonate: AP (lateral decubitus)					
Infant: AP (lateral decubitus)					
Child: AP (lateral decubitus)					

2. Adequate contrast resolution is present on chest projections when which lung structures are clearly demonstrated?

A. _____   D. _____

B. _____   E. _____

C. _____

3. Indicate whether the following statements are true (T) or false (F) as they relate to chest devices, tubes, and catheters by placing a T or F in front of the statement.

_____ A. It is within the technologist's scope of practice to immediately inform the radiologist or attending physician when a mispositioned device, line, or catheter is suspected.

_____ B. The endotracheal tube (ETT) is used to inflate the lung.

_____ C. For adults, the ETT should be positioned 3 to 5 inches (8 to 13 cm) superior to the tracheal bifurcation.

_____ D. The ETT should reside at the level of T4 on the neonate.

_____ E. With head rotation and cervical vertebrae flexion and extension, the ETT tip can move superiorly and inferiorly.

_____ F. The pleural drainage tube is used to remove fluid or air from the lung cavity.

_____ G. For drainage of fluid, the pleural drainage tube is placed laterally at the level of the fifth or sixth intercostal space.

_____ H. A central venous catheter (CVC) is used to allow infusion of substances too toxic for peripheral infusion.

_____ I. Projections taken for CVC placement should visualize the CVC tip extending to the superior vena cava.

_____ J. The pulmonary arterial catheter (PAC) measures atrial pressures, pulmonary artery pressures, and cardiac output.

_____ K. The PAC tip should rest in the superior vena cava.

_____ L. An umbilical artery catheter (UAC) is found in neonates and is used to measure oxygen saturation.

_____ M. An umbilical vein catheter (UVC) is used to deliver fluids and medications.

_____ N. The UVC is radiographically seen on lateral chest projections running adjacent to the vertebral bodies.

_____ O. A pacemaker is used to regulate the heart rate by supplying electrical stimulation to the heart.

_____ P. Lifting the patient's arm whose pacemaker was inserted within 24 hours of the examination may cause the pacemaker and catheter to dislodge.

_____ Q. The automatic implantable cardioverter defibrillator (ICD) is used to detect arrhythmias and deliver an electrical shock to the heart.

4. Identify the internal tube or line demonstrated in the following projections.

Figure 3-2

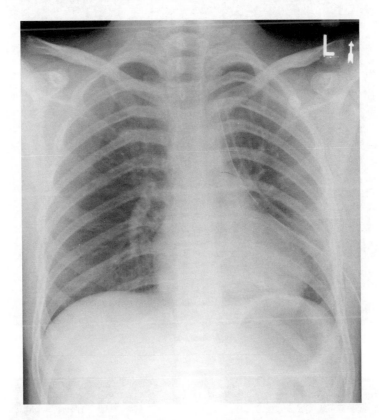

A. Figure 3-2: _____

Figure 3-3

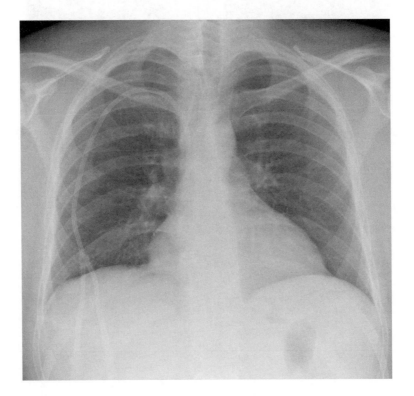

B. Figure 3-3: _____

Chapter **3 Image Analysis of the Chest and Abdomen**

Figure 3-4

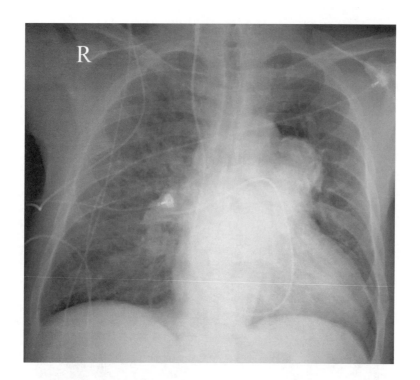

C. Figure 3-4:_____

Figure 3-5

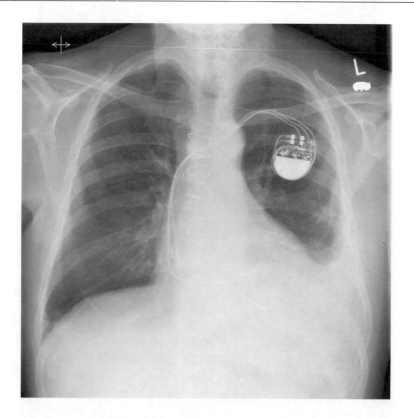

D. Figure 3-5:_____

5. Match the term with its definition.

_____ A. Pleural cavity   1. Density line created when fluid and air separate

_____ B. Pneumothorax   2. Spinous process of the seventh cervical vertebra

_____ C. Pneumectomy   3. Within the abdominal cavity

_____ D. Intraperitoneal   4. Cavity encasing the lungs

_____ E. Vertebra prominens   5. Removal of lung

_____ F. Apex (apical)   6. Air in pleural cavity

_____ G. Air-fluid line   7. Narrow end of a cone-shaped object

6. How must the patient and CR be positioned for a PA chest projection to obtain the most accurate assessment of air-fluid levels in the thorax?

A. Patient: _____

B. CR: _____

7. Identify the pathological condition demonstrated in the following projections.

Figure 3-6

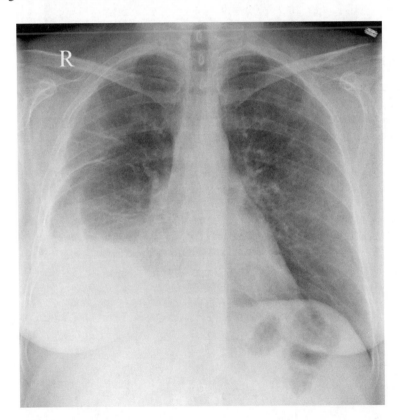

A. Right inferior lung (Figure 3-6)

_____

Figure 3-7

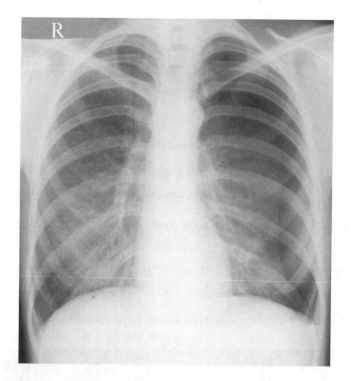

B. Left superior and lateral lung (Figure 3-7)

Figure 3-8

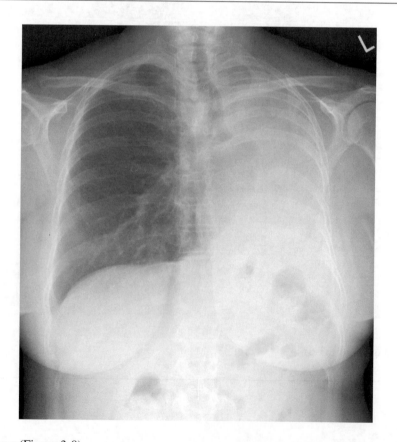

C. Left inferior lung (Figure 3-8)

8. Identify which body habitus type is being demonstrated in each of the following projections.

Figure 3-9

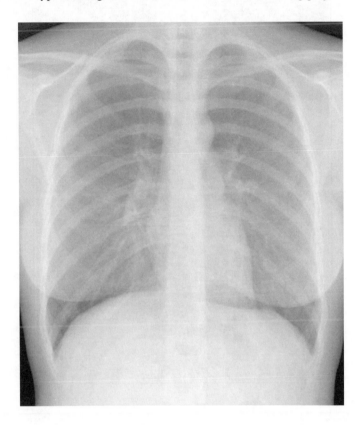

A. Figure 3-9:_____

Figure 3-10

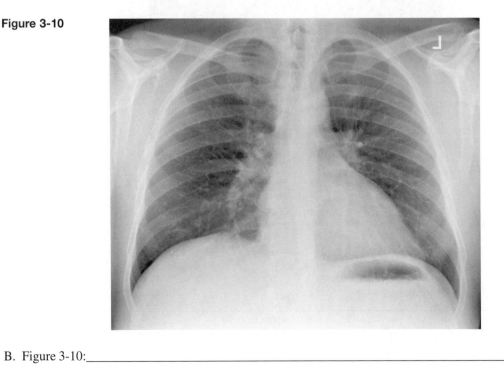

B. Figure 3-10:_____

Figure 3-11

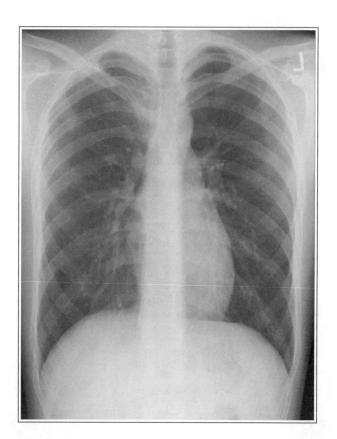

C. Figure 3-11: _____

Figure 3-12

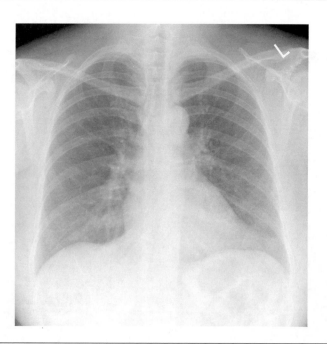

D. Figure 3-12: _____

PA Projection

9. Complete the statements below referring to adult PA chest projection analysis guidelines.

PA Chest Projection Analysis Guidelines

- The (A) _____ thoracic vertebra is at the center of the exposure field.

- Both lungs, from apices to (B) _____, are included within the collimated field.

- Distances from the vertebral column to the sternal clavicular ends are (C) _____, and lengths of the right and left corresponding posterior ribs are equal.

- Clavicles are positioned on the same (D) _____ plane.

- Scapulae are located (E) _____ the lung field.

- Manubrium is superimposed by the (F) _____ vertebra, with 1 inch (2.5 cm) of apical lung field visible above the clavicles.

- At least (G) _____ posterior ribs are visualized above the diaphragm.

Figure 3-13

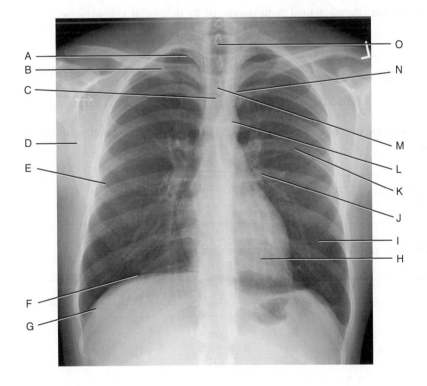

10. Identify the labeled anatomy on the PA chest projection in Figure 3-13.

A. _____   E. _____

B. _____   F. _____

C. _____   G. _____

D. _____   H. _____

Chapter **3** **Image Analysis of the Chest and Abdomen**

I. _____   M. _____

J. _____   N. _____

K. _____   O. _____

L. _____

11. List the three dimensions in which the lungs expand and contract during inspiration and expiration.

    A. _____

    B. _____

    C. _____

12. The _____ dimension of the thorax expands the most during inspiration.

13. List two situations that could prevent full lung expansion during the taking of chest projections.

    A. _____

    B. _____

14. What body type requires the computed radiography IR to be placed crosswise when a PA chest projection is taken?

    A. _____

    Describe the lung shape of such a patient.

    B. _____

15. What body types will require the exposure field to be open more in the lengthwise dimension when a PA chest projection is taken?

    A. _____

    Describe the lung shapes of such patients.

    B. _____

16. State how the patient is positioned to prevent rotation on a PA chest projection.

    _____

    _____

Figure 3-14

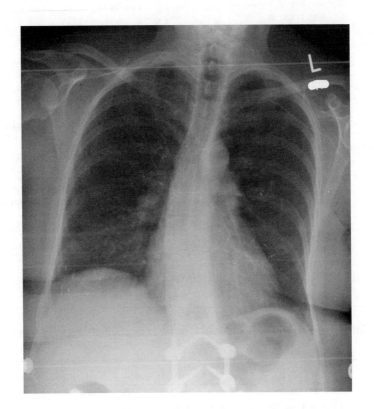

17. A. What spinal condition is demonstrated in the PA chest projection in Figure 3-14?

    _____

   B. Can patient positioning be adjusted to offset this rotated appearance on such a patient?

    _____

   C. How can this condition be distinguished from rotation on a PA chest projection?

    _____

18. How is the patient positioned to place the clavicles on the same horizontal plane on a PA chest projection?

    _____

19. How is the patient positioned for a PA chest projection to place the scapulae outside the lung field?

    _____

20. The level at which the manubrium is visible on the vertebral column and the amount of apical lung field demonstrated above the clavicles are determined by the tilt of the patient's (A) _____ plane. When this plane is vertical, the manubrium will be at the level of the (B) _____ thoracic vertebra, and approximately (C) _____ inch(es) of the apices will be demonstrated above the clavicles.

Chapter **3** **Image Analysis of the Chest and Abdomen**

21. On an accurately positioned PA chest projection, the clavicles should be horizontal. Which two aspects of the setup procedure can be mispositioned to result in somewhat vertically running clavicles?

A. _____

B. _____

22. Why will an increase in lung aeration be obtained when a PA chest projection is taken with the patient in an upright position versus a supine or seated position? _____

_____

23. What two positioning procedures will provide a PA chest projection with the greatest amount of vertical lung field?

A. _____

B. _____

24. Why are chest projections exposed after the patient has taken the second full inspiration?

_____

25. List two patient conditions that may indicate the need for an expiration chest projection to be taken.

A. _____

B. _____

26. On an expiration PA chest projection, the diaphragm will be positioned (A) _____ (higher/lower), fewer than (B) _____ posterior ribs will be demonstrated above the diaphragm, and the heart shadow will appear (C) _____ and (D) _____.

27. For an accurately positioned PA chest projection, a(n) (A) _____ CR is centered to the (B) _____ plane at a level approximately 8 inches (20 cm) inferior to the (C) _____.

28. For a right AP oblique (RPO) chest projection, which side of the thorax will be best demonstrated? _____

_____

For the following descriptions of PA chest projections with poor positioning, state how the patient would have been mispositioned for such a projection to result.

29. Whereas the vertebral column is superimposed over the right sternoclavicular (SC) joint, the left SC joint is demonstrated without vertebral superimposition.

_____

30. The clavicles are not positioned on the same horizontal plane. The lateral clavicular ends are elevated. The manubrium is at the same level as the fourth thoracic vertebra.

_____

31. The right scapula is demonstrated within the lung field.

_____

32. The clavicles are horizontal, the manubrium is situated at the level of the fifth thoracic vertebra, and more than 1 inch (2.5 cm) of the chest apex is demonstrated superior to the clavicles.

_____

For the following PA chest projections with poor positioning, state which anatomic structures are misaligned and how the patient should be repositioned for an optimal projection to be obtained.

Figure 3-15

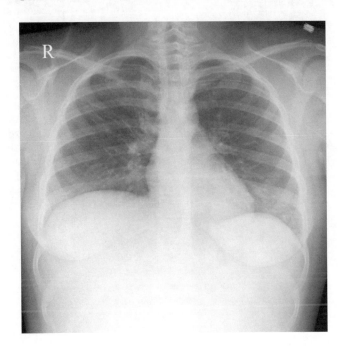

33. Figure 3-15:

_____

_____

Figure 3-16

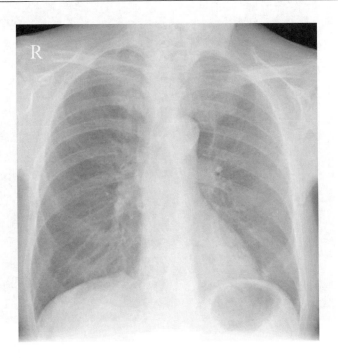

34. Figure 3-16:

_____

_____

Figure 3-17

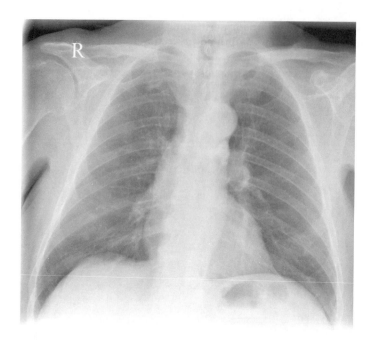

35. Figure 3-17:

_____

_____

Figure 3-18

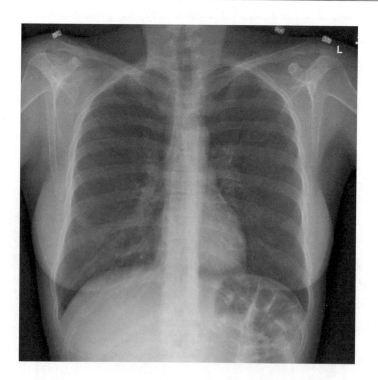

36. Figure 3-18:

_____

_____

Figure 3-19

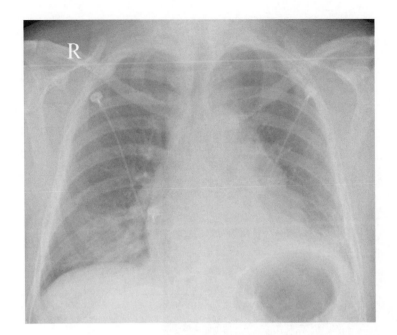

37. Figure 3-19:

_____

_____

Figure 3-20

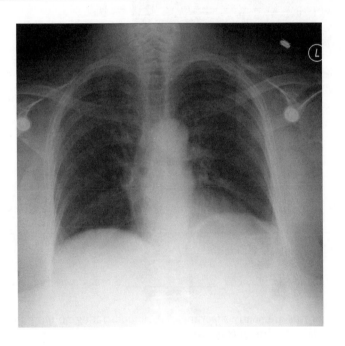

38. Figure 3-20:

_____

_____

Lateral Projection

39. Identify the labeled anatomy in Figure 3-21.

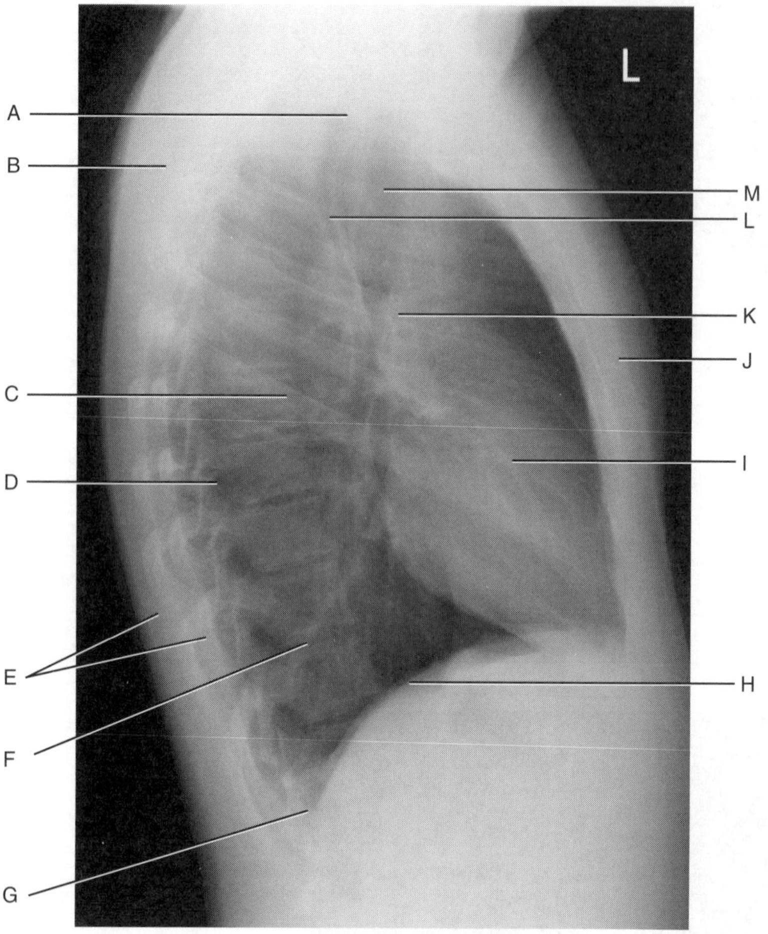

Figure 3-21

A. _____

B. _____

C. _____

D. _____

E. _____

F. _____

G. _____

H. _____

I. _____

J. _____

K. _____

L. _____

M. _____

40. Complete the statements below referring to lateral chest projection analysis guidelines.

Lateral Chest Projection Analysis Guidelines

- Midcoronal plane, at the level of the (A) _____ thoracic vertebra, is at the center of the exposure field.

- Right and left posterior ribs are nearly superimposed, demonstrating no more than a (B) _____ of space between them, and the sternum is in profile.

- Lungs are demonstrated without foreshortening, with nearly superimposed (C) _____

- No humeral soft tissue is seen superimposing the (D) _____ lung apices.

- Anteroinferior lung and heart shadows are well defined.

- Hemidiaphragms demonstrate a gentle, superiorly bowed contour and are inferior to the (E) _____ thoracic vertebra.

41. How is the patient positioned to prevent rotation on a lateral chest projection?

_____

42. Which side of the thorax will demonstrate the greatest magnification when a left lateral chest projection is taken?

   A. _____

   Explain your answer.
   B. _____

43. How is rotation identified on a lateral chest projection?

44. List three methods that can be used to identify the right and left hemidiaphragms on a lateral chest projection with poor positioning.

   A. _____

   B. _____

   C. _____

45. Which side of the chest cavity contains most of the heart? _____

46. A rotated lateral chest projection demonstrates the left lung posteriorly, with 2.5 inches (6.25 cm) of space between the posterior ribs. How should the patient be adjusted, and how much movement from the original position should

   be made? _____

_____

47. State a method of distinguishing scoliosis from rotation on a lateral chest projection.

_____

_____

48. How is the patient positioned with respect to the IR for a lateral chest projection to prevent lung foreshortening?

_____

_____

49. Which lung and diaphragm are situated higher on most patients? _____

50. List two expected differences that would be demonstrated between a right and a left lateral chest projection.

   A. _____

   _____

   B. _____

   _____

51. State whether it is best to take a right or left lateral chest projection for the following.

   A. To evaluate right lung details: _____

   B. To evaluate the heart: _____

52. How is the patient positioned for a lateral chest projection to prevent the humeral soft tissue from being superimposed over the anterior lung apices?

_____

53. How can one determine if full lung aeration has occurred for a lateral chest projection?

_____

54. What two positioning procedures will provide a lateral chest projection with the greatest amount of vertical lung field?

A. _____

B. _____

55. Which thoracic vertebra has the last rib attached to it? _____

56. To accurately center the chest on a lateral chest projection, the CR is centered to the (A) _____ plane at a level 9 inches (23 cm) (B) _____ to the vertebral prominens.

57. Which anatomic structures are included in a lateral chest projection for which the subject was accurately positioned?

_____

_____

For the following descriptions of left lateral chest projections with poor positioning, state how the patient would have been mispositioned for such a projection to result.

58. The humeri soft tissue shadows are superimposed over the anterior lung apices.

_____

59. The posterior ribs are separated by more than 0.5 inch (1.25 cm), and the superior heart shadow is seen extending beyond the sternum into the anteriorly situated lung.

_____

60. One hemidiaphragm is demonstrated superior to the other, and the gastric bubble is situated beneath the superior hemidiaphragm.

_____

For the following lateral chest projections with poor positioning, state which anatomic structures are misaligned and how the patient should be repositioned for an optimal projection to be obtained.

Figure 3-22

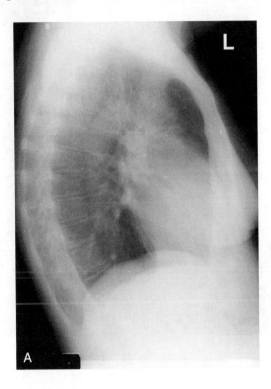

61. Figure 3-22: _____

_____

Figure 3-23

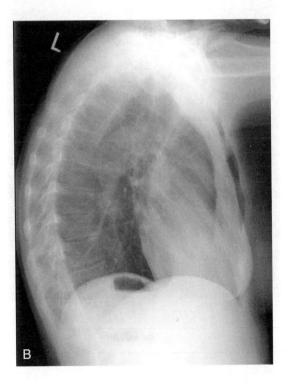

62. Figure 3-23: _____

_____

Figure 3-24

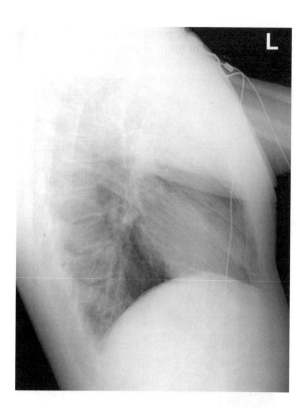

63. Figure 3-24: _____

_____

Figure 3-25

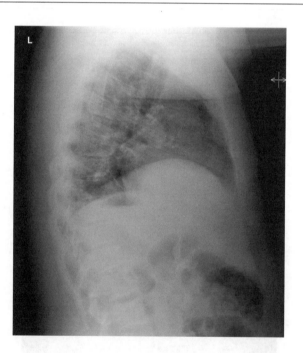

64. Figure 3-25: _____

_____

The following chest case study includes PA and lateral chest projections from the same patient. Evaluate the projections for accurate positioning.

Figure 3-26

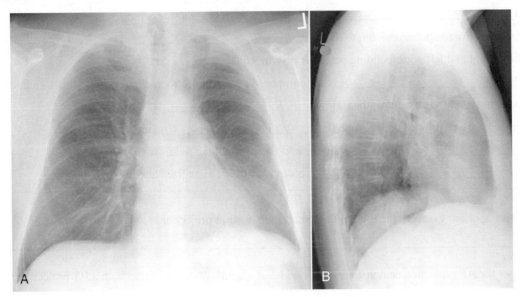

65. Figure 3-26:

    A. _____

    B. _____

AP Projection (Supine or With Mobile X-Ray Unit)

66. Identify the labeled anatomy in Figure 3-27.

Figure 3-27

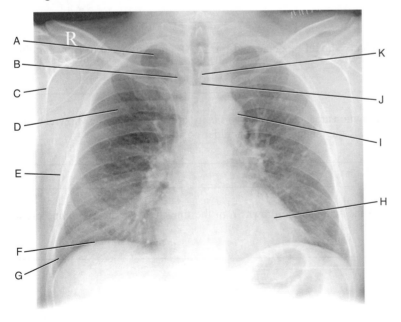

    A. _____

    B. _____

    C. _____

    D. _____

    E. _____

    F. _____

    G. _____

    H. _____

    I. _____

    J. _____

    K. _____

Chapter **3 Image Analysis of the Chest and Abdomen**

67. Complete the statements below referring to adult AP chest projection analysis guidelines.

AP Chest (Supine or Mobile) Projection Analysis Guidelines
■ (A) _____ thoracic vertebra is at the center of the exposure field.
■ Distances from vertebral column to (B) _____ are equal, and lengths of the right and left corresponding posterior ribs are equal.
■ (C) _____ is superimposed by the fourth thoracic vertebra, with 1 inch (2.5 cm) of apical lung field visible above the (D) _____ .
■ Clavicles are positioned on the same (E) _____ plane when possible.
■ (F) _____ are located outside the lung field, when possible.
■ (G) _____ posterior ribs are visualized above the diaphragm.

68. Why is it important to record the time of day on all mobile chest projections?

_____

69. Why does the AP projection demonstrate increased heart magnification compared with a PA projection?

_____

70. Why are air-fluid levels undetectable when the patient is supine?

_____

71. State how the patient is positioned to prevent rotation on an AP chest projection.

_____

72. How can rotation be identified on an AP chest projection?

_____

73. When the patient's condition allows, the shoulders should be depressed for an AP chest projection. How can this movement be identified on the projection?

_____

74. When an AP chest projection is obtained that demonstrates somewhat vertically appearing clavicles, how can one determine if this appearance is a result of poor CR alignment or poor shoulder positioning?

_____

_____

75. When the patient's condition allows, how can the scapulae be drawn from the lung field on an AP supine chest projection?

_____

76. Poor CR alignment on a mobile chest projection will affect the amount of apical lung field demonstrated superior to the clavicles and the contour of the posterior ribs. For each of the following situations, describe the expected change in apical lung visualization and posterior rib contour.

A. The CR was angled too caudally.

_____

B. The CR was angled too cephalically.

_____

77. How can the CR be adjusted to improve the posterior rib contour and eliminate superimposition of the chin on the apices when imaging a kyphotic patient for an AP chest projection?

_____

78. Why is a 5-degree caudal CR angle used for supine AP chest projections?

_____

79. Why are fewer posterior ribs demonstrated above the diaphragm on a supine AP chest projection than on an upright PA chest projection?

_____

80. How is the patient instructed to breathe to obtain maximum lung aeration?

_____

81. Accurate centering on an AP chest projection is accomplished by centering the CR to the (A) _____

plane at a level (B) _____ inches inferior to the (C) _____.

82. Which anatomic structures are included on an accurately positioned AP chest projection?

_____

For the following descriptions of AP chest projections with poor positioning, state how the patient would have been mispositioned or the CR misaligned for such a projection to result.

83. The left SC joint is visible away from the vertebral column, and the right SC joint is superimposed over the vertebral column (list both the patient and CR mispositioning that could cause this projection).

_____

_____

84. The manubrium is shown superimposed over the fifth thoracic vertebra with more than 1 inch (2.5 cm) of the apical lung field visible above the clavicles, and the posterior ribs demonstrate a vertical contour.

_____

_____

85. The manubrium is shown superimposed over the third vertebra with less than 1 inch (2.5 cm) of apical lung field visible above the clavicles, and the posterior ribs demonstrate a horizontal contour.

_____

_____

86. A projection of a patient with severe kyphosis demonstrates the chin superimposed over the apical region, and the posterior ribs demonstrate a vertical contour.

_____

_____

For the following AP chest projections with poor positioning, state which anatomic structures are misaligned and how the patient should be repositioned for an optimal projection to be obtained.

Figure 3-28

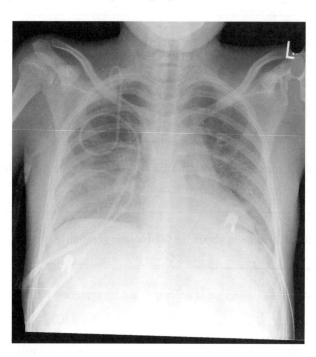

87. Figure 3-28:

_____

_____

Figure 3-29

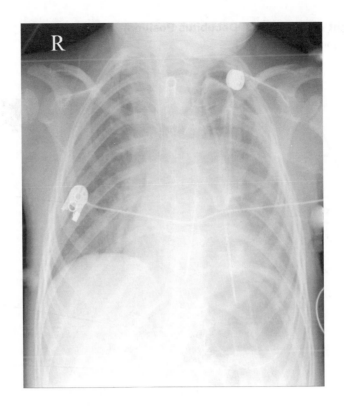

88. Figure 3-29:

_____

_____

Figure 3-30

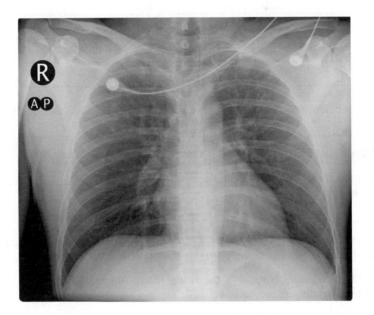

89. Figure 3-30:

_____

_____

AP or PA Projection (Right or Left Lateral Decubitus Position)

90. Identify the labeled anatomy in Figure 3-31.

Figure 3-31

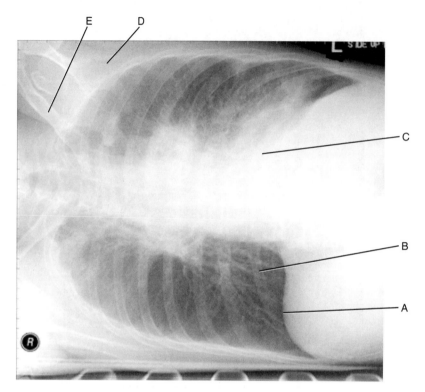

A. _____

B. _____

C. _____

D. _____

E. _____

91. Complete the statements below referring to adult AP/PA decubitus chest projection analysis guidelines.

AP/PA (Lateral Decubitus) Projection Analysis Guidelines
■ Arrow or "word" marker identifies the side of the patient positioned (A) _____ from the imaging table or cart.
■ (B) _____ thoracic vertebra is at the center of the exposure field.
■ Distances from the (C) _____ to the sternal clavicular ends are equal, and lengths of the right and left corresponding posterior ribs are equal.
■ The arms, mandible, and lateral borders of the scapulae are situated (D) _____, and lateral aspects of the clavicles are projected upward.
■ The manubrium is superimposed by the (E) _____ vertebra.
■ At the least nine posterior ribs are visualized above the (F) _____.

92. The AP/PA (decubitus) projection is primarily performed to confirm the presence of (A) _____ or (B) _____ levels within the pleural cavity.

93. If fluid is present within the pleural cavity on an AP/PA (decubitus) chest projection, where will it be located?

_____

94. For each situation below, state whether a right or left AP/PA decubitus chest projection should be taken.

    A. Right pneumothorax: _____

    B. Left pleural effusion: _____

95. To avoid rotation on AP/PA (decubitus) chest projections, align the patient's (A) _____, (B) _____, and (C) _____ perpendicular to the cart.

96. Will an AP or PA (decubitus) chest projection demonstrate the sixth and seventh cervical vertebrae without distortion and open intervertebral disk space?

_____

97. The lateral scapular borders are situated outside the lung field when the arms are positioned _____ for an AP/PA (decubitus) chest projection.

98. Chest foreshortening can be avoided on an AP/PA (decubitus) chest projection by positioning the (A) _____ plane (B) _____ (perpendicular/parallel) to the IR.

99. How can the patient be positioned for an AP/PA (decubitus) chest projection to prevent the cart pad from creating an artifact line along the lung field positioned against it?

_____

_____

For the following descriptions of AP/PA (decubitus) chest projections with poor positioning, state how the patient would have been positioned for such a projection to be obtained.

100. Whereas an AP (decubitus) chest projection demonstrates the right SC joint superimposed over the vertebral column, the left SC joint does not demonstrate vertebral superimposition.

_____

101. An AP decubitus chest projection demonstrates the manubrium at the level of the second thoracic vertebra.

_____

For the following AP/PA (decubitus) chest projections with poor positioning, state which anatomic structures are misaligned and how the patient should be repositioned for an optimal projection to be obtained.

Figure 3-32

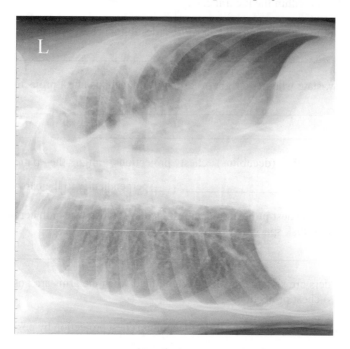

102. Figure 3-32, AP projection:

_____

_____

Figure 3-33

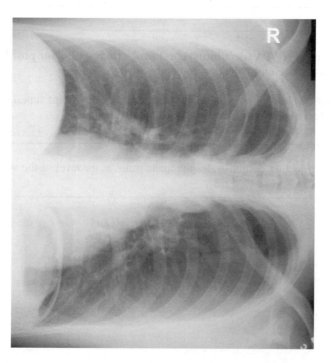

103. Figure 3-33, AP projection:

_____

_____

AP Axial Projection (Lordotic Position)

104. Identify the labeled anatomy in Figure 3-34.

Figure 3-34

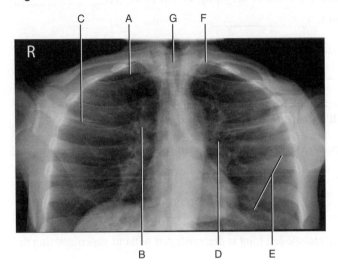

A. _____

B. _____

C. _____

D. _____

E. _____

F. _____

G. _____

105. Complete the statements below referring to adult AP axial (lordotic) chest projection analysis guidelines.

AP Axial (Lordotic) Chest Projection Analysis Guidelines
■ (A) _____ lung field is at the center of the exposure field.
■ Sternal clavicular ends of clavicles are projected (B) _____ to the lung apices, and posterior and anterior aspects of the first through fourth ribs lie (C) _____ and are superimposed.
■ Distances from (D) _____ to the sternal clavicular ends are equal.

106. The AP axial chest projection is taken to visualize the _____.

107. Describe three methods that can be used to position the clavicles superior to the lung apices.

A. _____

_____

B. _____

_____

C. _____

_____

108. An AP axial chest projection with poor positioning demonstrates the clavicles superimposed over the lung apices. Which two positional changes can be made to obtain a projection with accurate positioning?

A. _____

B. _____

109. How can rotation be identified on an AP axial chest projection?

_____

110. An accurately centered AP axial chest projection is accomplished by centering the CR to the (A) _____

plane halfway between the (B) _____ and (C) _____.

111. Which anatomic structures are included on an AP axial chest projection with accurate positioning?

_____

For the following descriptions of AP axial chest projections with poor positioning, state how the patient would have been mispositioned or the CR misaligned for such a projection to be obtained.

112. The clavicles are superimposed over the lung apices, and the anterior ribs appear inferior to their corresponding posterior ribs.

_____

_____

113. The right SC joint superimposes the vertebral column, and the left joint is demonstrated without superimposing the vertebral column.

_____

_____

For the following lordotic chest projection with poor positioning, state which anatomic structures are misaligned and how the patient should be repositioned for an optimal projection to be obtained.

Figure 3-35

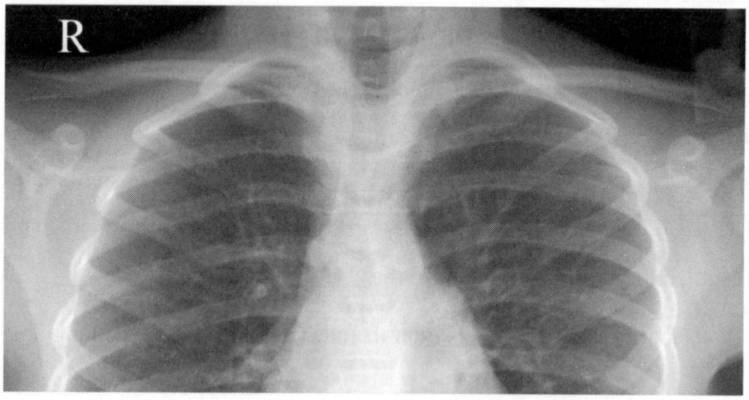

114. Figure 3-35:

_____

_____

Pediatric Chest

115. Why do neonatal and infant chest projections demonstrate less contrast than adult chest projections?

_____

116. Discuss the importance of the neonate's or infant's face being positioned forward.

_____

Neonate and Infant: AP Projection (Supine or With Mobile X-Ray Unit)

117. Identify the labeled anatomy in Figure 3-36.

Figure 3-36

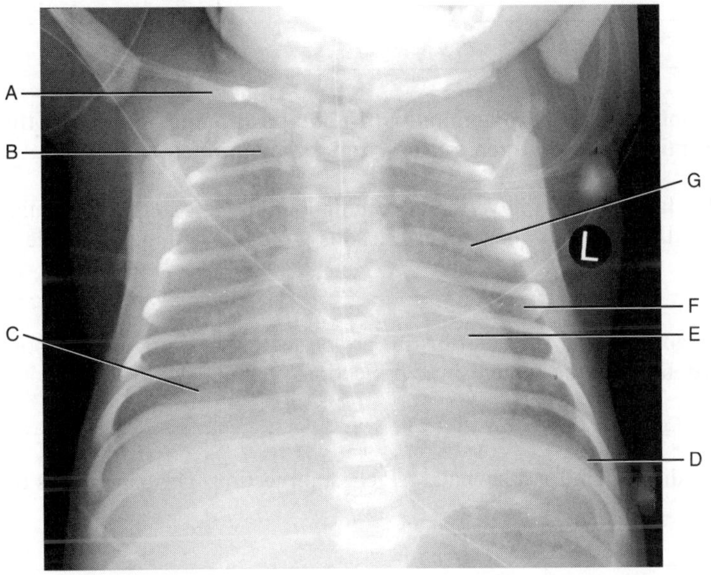

A. _____

B. _____

C. _____

D. _____

E. _____

F. _____

G. _____

118. Complete the statements below referring to neonate and infant AP chest projection analysis guidelines.

Neonate and Infant AP Chest Projection Analysis Guidelines
■ (A) _____ thoracic vertebra is at the center of the exposure field.
■ Distances from the vertebral column to the sternal ends of the clavicles are (B) _____, and the lengths of the right and left corresponding posterior ribs are (C) _____.
■ When a 5-degree caudal CR angle is used, the anterior ribs are projecting (D) _____, and the posterior ribs demonstrate a gentle, (E) _____ bowed contour.
■ Neonate: (F) _____ posterior ribs are demonstrated above the diaphragm, and the lungs demonstrate a fluffy appearance with linear-appearing connecting tissue.
■ Infant: (G) _____ posterior ribs are demonstrated above the diaphragm.
■ (H) _____ does not obscure the airway or apical lung field.

119. Accurate centering is seen on neonatal or infant AP chest projections when a perpendicular CR is centered to the (A) _____ plane at the level of the (B) _____. The (C) _____ _____ should be included on the projection.

120. What causes the lungs on a neonatal chest projection to have a fluffy appearance?

_____

121. Explain when the projection should be exposed in the following situations to obtain maximum lung expansion.

A. Neonate breathing without a ventilator: _____

_____

B. Neonate on a high-frequency ventilator: _____

_____

For the following descriptions of neonatal or infant AP chest projections with poor positioning, state how the patient would have been mispositioned or the CR misaligned for such a projection to be obtained.

122. The right sternal clavicular end is demonstrated farther from the vertebral column than the left sternal clavicular end, and the right lower posterior ribs are longer than the left. The patient's head is turned toward the right side.

_____

123. The chest demonstrates an excessively lordotic appearance. The anterior ribs are projecting upward, and the posterior ribs are horizontal. The sixth thoracic vertebra is at the center of the projection.

_____

124. Seven posterior ribs are demonstrated above the diaphragm for a neonatal AP chest projection. The patient was on a conventional ventilator.

_____

125. The patient's mandible is superimposed over the airway and apical lung field.

_____

For the following AP neonatal or infant chest projections with poor positioning, state which anatomic structures are misaligned and how the patient should be repositioned for an optimal projection to be obtained.

Figure 3-37

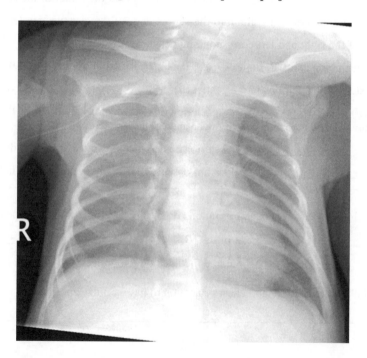

126. Figure 3-37:

_____

_____

Figure 3-38

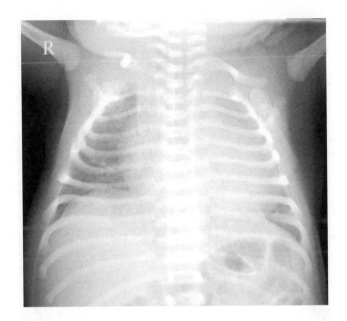

127. Figure 3-38:

_____

_____

Figure 3-39

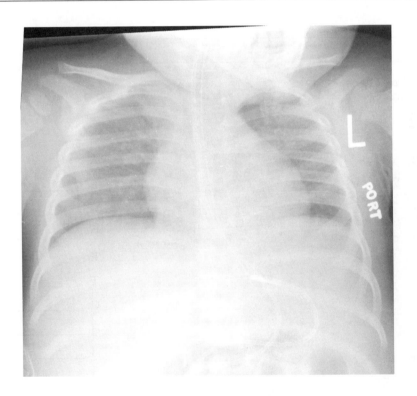

128. Figure 3-39:

_____

_____

Figure 3-40

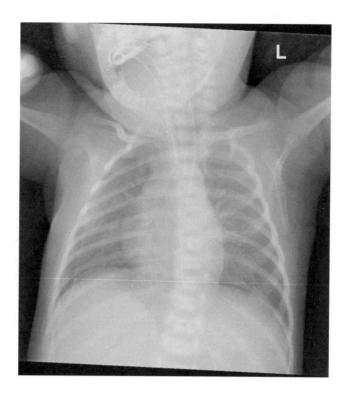

129. Figure 3-40:

_____

_____

Child: PA and AP Projections

130. Identify the labeled anatomy in Figure 3-41.

Figure 3-41

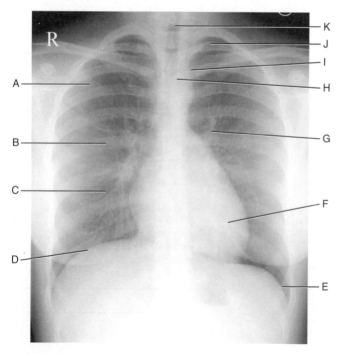

A. _____

B. _____

C. _____

D. _____

E. _____

F. _____

G. _____

H. _____

I. _____

J. _____

K. _____

For the following descriptions of child PA/AP chest projections with poor positioning, state how the patient would have been mispositioned or the central ray misaligned for such a projection to be obtained.

131. Mobile AP projection: The left sternoclavicular end is visualized without vertebral column superimposition, and the vertebral column is superimposed over the right sternal clavicular end.

_____

_____

132. PA projection: Six posterior ribs are demonstrated above the diaphragm.

_____

_____

133. Mobile AP projection: The manubrium is superimposed over the fifth thoracic vertebra, the posterior ribs demonstrate vertical contour, and more than 1 inch (2.5 cm) of apical lung field is visible above the clavicles.

_____

_____

134. PA projection: The second thoracic vertebra is superimposed over the manubrium.

_____

_____

135. PA projection: The fourth thoracic vertebra is superimposed over the manubrium, and the lateral ends of the clavicles are projecting superiorly.

_____

_____

For the following PA/AP child chest projections with poor positioning, state which anatomic structures are misaligned and how the patient should be repositioned for an optimal projection to be obtained.

Figure 3-42

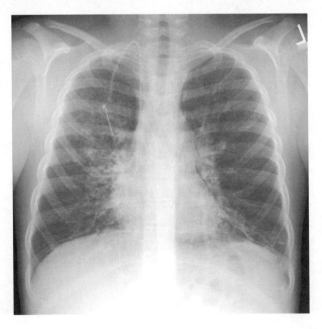

136. Figure 3-42, PA projection:

_____

_____

Figure 3-43

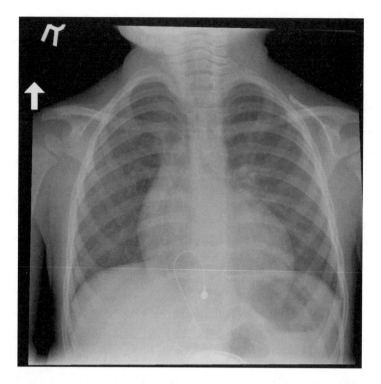

137. Figure 3-43, PA projection:

_____

_____

Figure 3-44

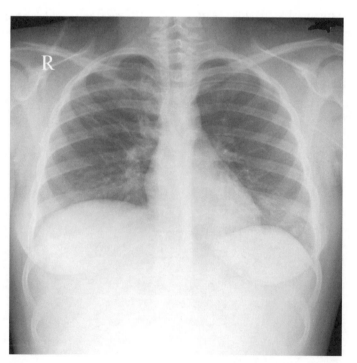

138. Figure 3-44, PA projection:

_____

_____

78

Figure 3-45

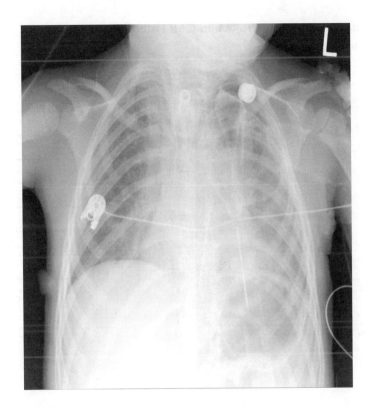

139. Figure 3-45, AP projection:

_____

_____

Figure 3-46

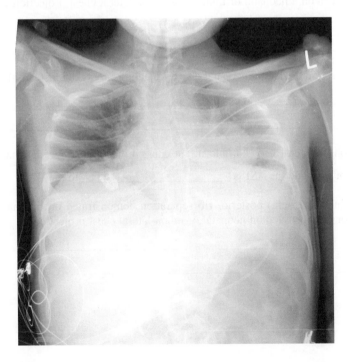

140. Figure 3-46, AP projection:

_____

_____

Chapter **3** **Image Analysis of the Chest and Abdomen**

Neonate and Infant: Cross-Table Lateral Projection (Left Lateral Position)

141. Identify the labeled anatomy in Figure 3-47.

Figure 3-47

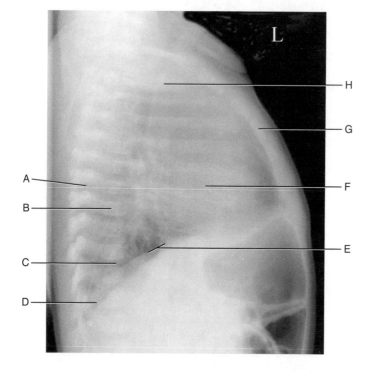

A. _____

B. _____

C. _____

D. _____

E. _____

F. _____

G. _____

H. _____

142. Accurate centering is seen on a neonatal or infant cross-table lateral chest projection when the CR is centered to the (A) _____ plane at the (B) _____. The (C) _____ should be included on the projection.

143. List two reasons why cross-table lateral neonatal chest projections are taken instead of overhead projections.

A. _____

B. _____

144. To avoid chest rotation on lateral neonatal and infant chest projections, align an imaginary line connecting the shoulders, the posterior ribs, and the ASISs _____ to the IR.

145. Explain why the 0.5-inch (1.25-cm) posterior rib separation demonstrated on optimally positioned adult lateral chest projections is not demonstrated on neonatal or infant lateral chest projections.

_____

_____

For the following descriptions of neonatal or infant lateral chest projections with poor positioning, state how the patient would have been mispositioned or the CR misaligned for such a projection to be obtained.

146. The left posterior ribs are demonstrated posterior to the right posterior ribs.

_____

_____

147. The humeral soft tissue is superimposed over the anterior lung apices.

_____

_____

148. The patient's chin is demonstrated within the collimated field.

_____

_____

149. The hemidiaphragms demonstrate an exaggerated cephalic curvature and are positioned high in the thorax.

_____

_____

For the following neonatal or infant lateral chest projections with poor positioning, state which anatomic structures are misaligned and how the patient should be repositioned for an optimal projection to be obtained.

Figure 3-48

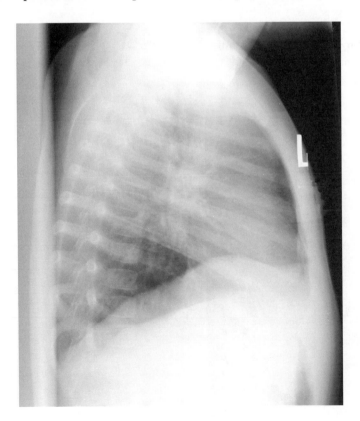

150. Figure 3-48:

_____

_____

Figure 3-49

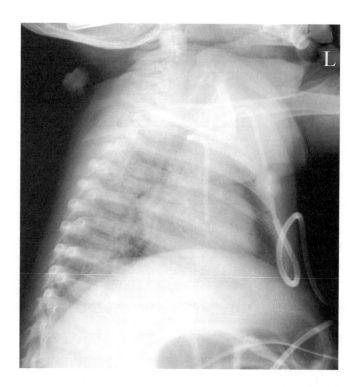

151. Figure 3-49:

_____

_____

Child: Lateral Projection (Left Lateral Position)

152. Identify the labeled anatomy in Figure 3-50.

Figure 3-50

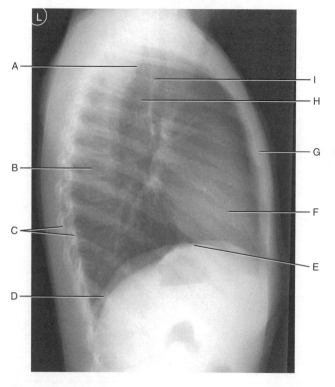

A. _____

B. _____

C. _____

D. _____

E. _____

F. _____

G. _____

H. _____

I. _____

For the following descriptions of child lateral chest projections with poor positioning, state how the patient would have been mispositioned or the CR misaligned for such a projection to be obtained.

153. More than 0.5 inch (1.25 cm) of separation is demonstrated between the posterior ribs. The gastric air bubble is adjacent to the posteriorly located lung.

   _____

   _____

154. The hemidiaphragms demonstrate an exaggerated cephalic curve, and they do not cover the entire 11th thoracic vertebra.

   _____

   _____

155. The humeral soft tissue is superimposed over the anterior lung apices.

   _____

   _____

For the following lateral child chest projections with poor positioning, state which anatomic structures are misaligned and how the patient should be repositioned for an optimal projection to be obtained.

Figure 3-51

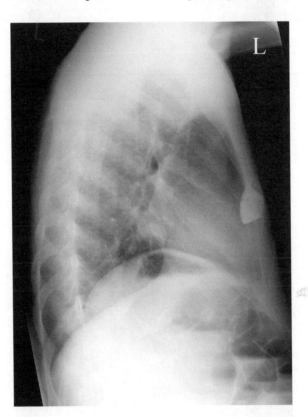

156. Figure 3-51:

   _____

   _____

Chapter **3** **Image Analysis of the Chest and Abdomen**

Figure 3-52

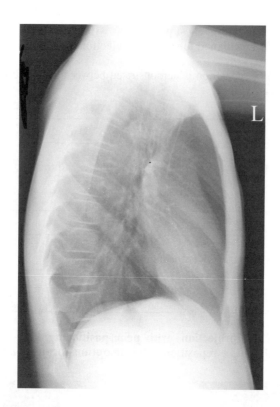

157. Figure 3-52:

_____

_____

Figure 3-53

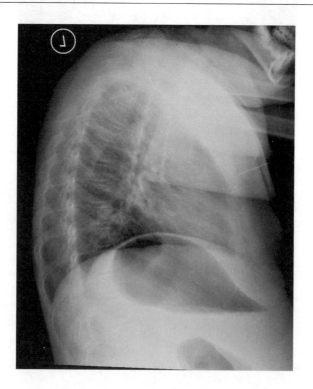

158. Figure 3-53:

_____

_____

Neonate and Infant: AP Projection (Right or Left Lateral Decubitus Projection)

159. Identify the labeled anatomy in Figure 3-54.

Figure 3-54

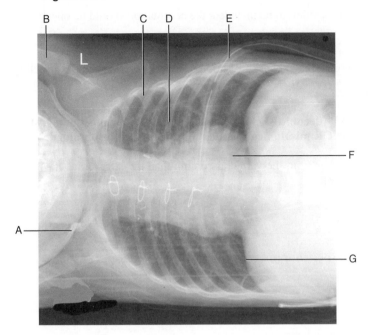

A. _____

B. _____

C. _____

D. _____

E. _____

F. _____

G. _____

160. Complete the statements below referring to neonate and infant AP (decubitus) chest projection analysis guidelines.

Neonate and Infant AP (Lateral Decubitus) Chest Projection Analysis Guidelines
■ (A) _____ thoracic vertebra is at the center of the exposure field.
■ Distances from the (B) _____ to the sternal ends of the clavicles are equal, and the lengths of the right and left corresponding posterior ribs are equal.
■ The chin and arms are situated outside the lung field, and the lateral aspects of the (C) _____ are projected upward.
■ With the posterior surface resting against IR, each upper anterior rib is demonstrated (D) _____ its corresponding posterior rib.
■ (E) _____ posterior ribs are demonstrated above the diaphragm, and the lungs demonstrate a fluffy appearance with linear-appearing connecting tissue.
■ Lung field positioned against the bed or cart is demonstrated without superimposition of the bed or cart pad.
■ (F) _____ plane is seen without lateral tilting.

161. To best demonstrate a pneumothorax on neonatal or infant AP (decubitus) chest projection, the affected side of the patient should be positioned

_____

162. For the upper airway on a neonatal or infant chest projection to be included, the collimation should be open to the

_____

163. To avoid chest rotation on a neonatal or infant AP (decubitus) chest projection, align an imaginary line connecting

the shoulders, the posterior ribs, and the ASISs _____ to the IR.

For the following descriptions of neonatal or infant AP (decubitus) chest projections with poor positioning, state how the patient would have been mispositioned or the CR misaligned for such a projection to be obtained.

164. The right sternal clavicular end is demonstrated farther from the vertebral column than the left sternal clavicular end, and the right posterior ribs are longer than the left.

_____

_____

165. The anterior ribs are projecting cephalically, and the posterior ribs are horizontal.

_____

_____

166. The six posterior ribs are demonstrated superior to the diaphragm.

_____

_____

167. The projection was taken to demonstrate pleural effusion on the right side. Artifact lines are superimposed over the lateral aspect of the right lung.

_____

_____

168. The projection was taken to demonstrate a right-side pneumothorax. The right arm is superimposed over the upper right lateral lung field.

_____

_____

For the following AP (decubitus) neonatal or infant chest projections with poor positioning, state which anatomic structures are misaligned and how the patient should be repositioned for an optimal projection to be obtained.

Figure 3-55

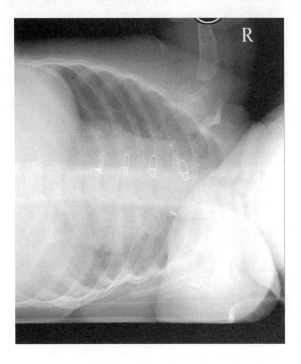

169. Figure 3-55:

_____

_____

Figure 3-56

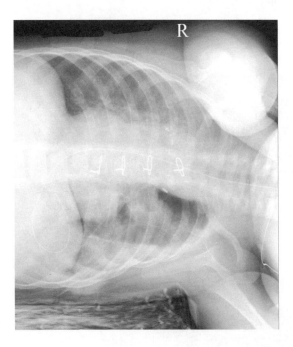

170. Figure 3-56:

_____

_____

Chapter **3 Image Analysis of the Chest and Abdomen**

Figure 3-57

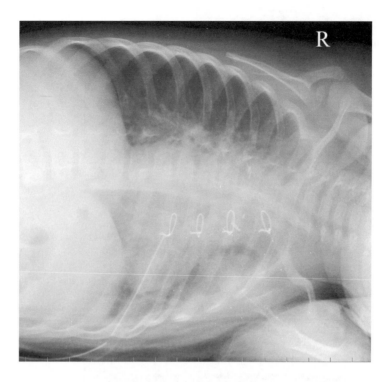

171. Figure 3-57:

_____

_____

Child Chest: AP or PA Projection (Right or Left Lateral Decubitus Position)

172. Identify the labeled anatomy in Figure 3-58.

Figure 3-58

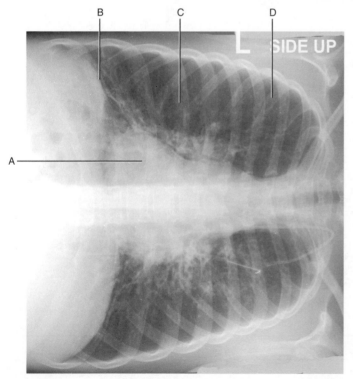

A. _____

B. _____

C. _____

D. _____

For the following descriptions of child AP/PA (decubitus) chest projections with poor positioning, state how the patient would have been mispositioned or the CR misaligned for such a projection to be obtained.

173. A PA (decubitus) chest projection demonstrates the vertebral column superimposed over the right SC joint.

_____

_____

174. Whereas an AP (decubitus) chest projection demonstrates the right SC joint superimposed over the vertebral column, the left SC joint does not demonstrate vertebral superimposition.

_____

_____

175. An AP (decubitus) chest projection demonstrates the manubrium at the level of the second thoracic vertebra.

_____

_____

For the following child AP (decubitus) chest projections with poor positioning, state which anatomic structures are misaligned and how the patient should be repositioned for an optimal projection to be obtained.

Figure 3-59

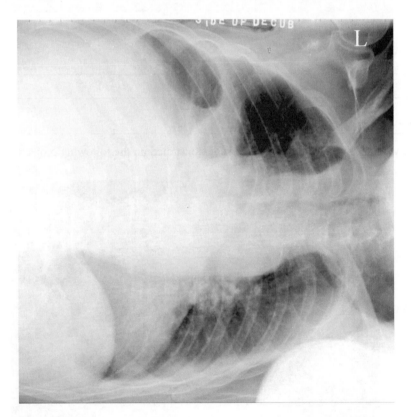

176. Figure 3-59:

_____

_____

Chapter **3 Image Analysis of the Chest and Abdomen**

Figure 3-60

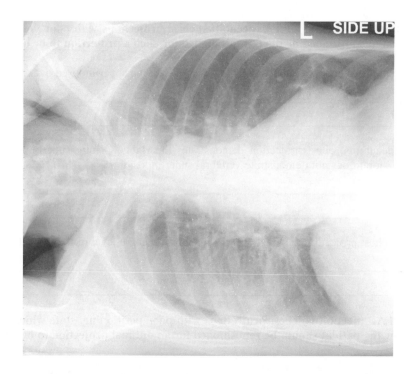

177. Figure 3-60:

_____

_____

ABDOMEN STUDY QUESTIONS

178. State whether voluntary or involuntary motion is demonstrated on the following projections.

Figure 3-61

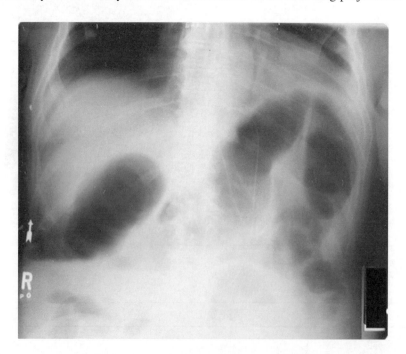

A. Figure 3-61: _____

Figure 3-62

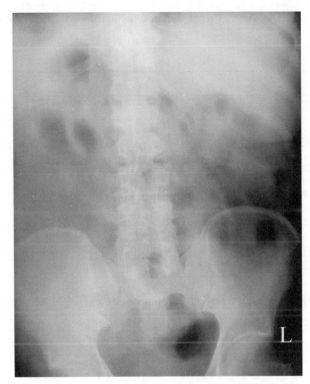

B. Figure 3-62: _____

179. Describe the location of the psoas major muscles.

_____

_____

180. A. Describe the location of the kidneys.

_____

   B. Which kidney is usually demonstrated inferiorly?

_____

   C. What causes the inferior location of this kidney?

_____

_____

181. List four anatomic structures that, when optimally demonstrated, ensure that the best possible technical data were used on AP abdominal projections.

   A. _____

   B. _____

   C. _____

   D. _____

182. State how the milliampere-seconds (mAs) or kV level is adjusted for AP abdominal projections of a patient who has a large amount of bowel gas.

   A. mAs: _____

   B. kV: _____

91

183. List four possible patient conditions that may require an increase in the routine exposure to obtain adequate IR exposure.

A. _____

B. _____

C. _____

D. _____

184. What can be done to avoid pendulous breasts from obscuring the upper abdominal area on an upright AP abdomen?

_____

185. Where is a nasogastric tube located in the abdomen when properly placed? _____

_____

186. Proper technical data have been used on neonatal and infant AP abdominal projections when which structures are visible on the projection? _____

187. Explain why abdominal organs are not well defined on neonatal and infant AP projections.

_____

_____

188. Complete Figure 3-63.

Figure 3-63

Adult Abdomen Technical Data					
Projection	kV	Grid	AEC	mAs	SID
AP, supine and upright					
AP (lateral decubitus)					
Pediatric Abdomen Technical Data					
Neonate: AP					
Infant: AP					
Child: AP					
Neonate: AP (lateral decubitus)					
Infant: AP (lateral decubitus)					
Child: AP (lateral decubitus)					

AP Projection (Supine and Upright)

189. Identify the labeled anatomy in Figure 3-64.

Figure 3-64

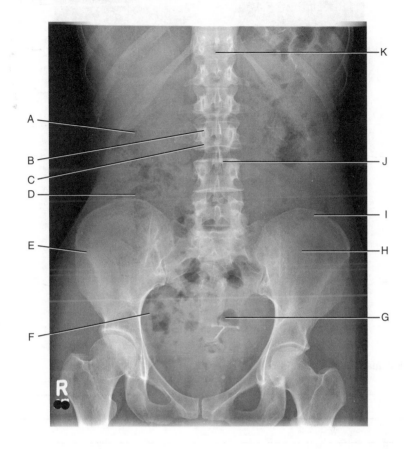

A. _____

B. _____

C. _____

D. _____

E. _____

F. _____

G. _____

H. _____

I. _____

J. _____

K. _____

Figure 3-65

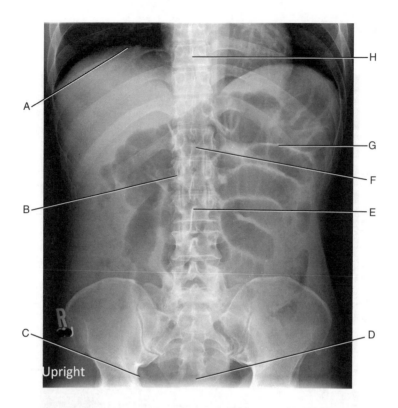

190. Identify the labeled anatomy in Figure 3-65.

A. _____

B. _____

C. _____

D. _____

E. _____

F. _____

G. _____

H. _____

191. Complete the statements below referring to adult AP abdomen projection analysis guidelines.

AP Abdomen Projection Analysis Guidelines

- Spinous processes are aligned with the midline of the (A) _____, and the distance from the pedicles to the spinous processes is the same on both sides. The sacrum is centered within the inlet of the pelvis and is aligned with the (B) _____.

- Diaphragm domes are located superior to the (C) _____ posterior ribs.

- Supine: (D) _____ lumbar vertebra is at the center of the exposure field.

- Upright: (E) _____ lumbar vertebra is at the center of the exposure field.

Figure 3-66

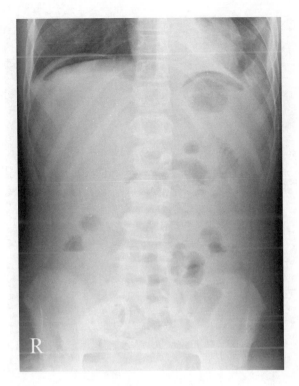

192. Identify the patient condition that is being demonstrated in Figure 3-66.

_____

193. Identify the body habitus demonstrated in the following figures.

Figure 3-67

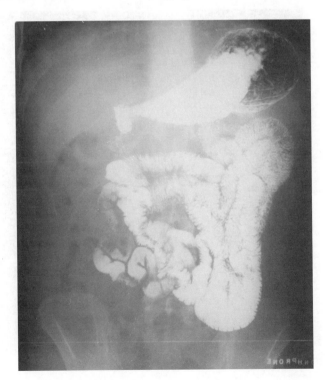

A. Figure 3-67:

_____

Figure 3-68

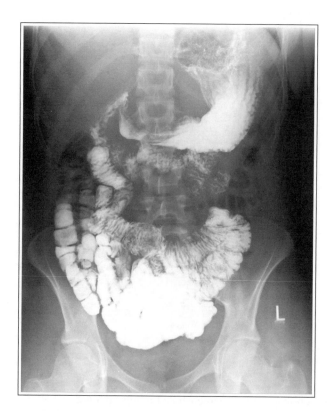

B. Figure 3-68:

Figure 3-69

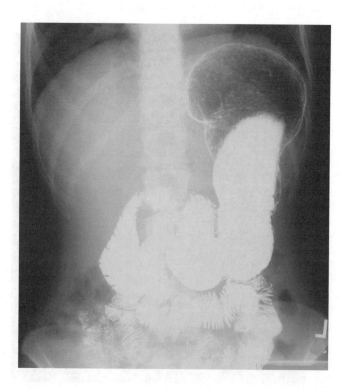

C. Figure 3-69:

194. How should the patient be positioned to prevent rotation on an AP abdominal projection?

_____

_____

195. A. To best demonstrate intraperitoneal air, how long should the patient be positioned upright before the projection is taken?

_____

B. Why is this time delay necessary?

_____

196. From full inspiration to expiration, the diaphragm position moves from a(n) (A) _____ (inferior/superior) to (B) _____ (inferior/superior) position. Whereas on full expiration the right side of the diaphragmatic dome will be at the same transverse level as the (C) _____ thoracic vertebra, on inspiration it is found at the (D) _____ thoracic vertebra.

197. A. What respiration is used for an AP abdominal projection?

_____

B. Why is this respiration used?

_____

198. State why it is important that both of the following structures are demonstrated on a supine abdominal projection.

A. 12th thoracic vertebrae:

_____

B. Pubis symphysis:

_____

199. Why is it necessary to center 1 inch (2.5 cm) more inferiorly on a male patient than a female patient to include the pubis symphysis?

_____

_____

200. Which anatomic structures are included on the following AP abdominal projections?

A. Supine: _____

B. Upright: _____

For the following descriptions of AP abdominal projections with poor positioning, state how the patient would have been mispositioned or the CR misaligned for such a projection to be obtained.

201. The distance from the right lumbar vertebral pedicles to the spinous processes is greater than the left pedicles to the spinous processes.

_____

_____

202. The upper abdominal region demonstrates an equal distance from the vertebral pedicles to the spinous processes on each side, and the lower abdominal region demonstrates the sacrum and pubis symphysis without alignment. The sacrum is rotated toward the right pelvic inlet.

_____

_____

203. The supine abdominal projection does not include the pubis symphysis or inferior peritoneal cavity.

_____

For the following AP abdominal projections with poor positioning, state which anatomic structures are misaligned and how the patient should be repositioned for an optimal projection to be obtained.

Figure 3-70

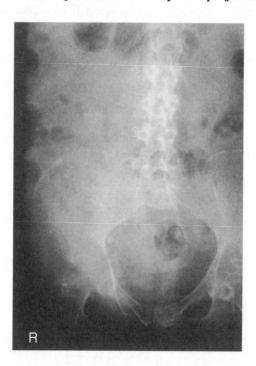

204. A supine abdominal projection was requested (Figure 3-70).

_____

_____

Figure 3-71

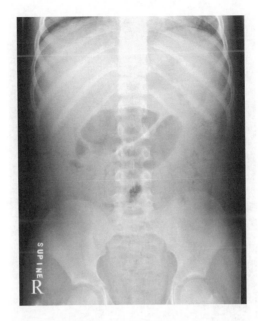

205. A supine abdominal projection was requested (Figure 3-71).

_____

_____

Figure 3-72

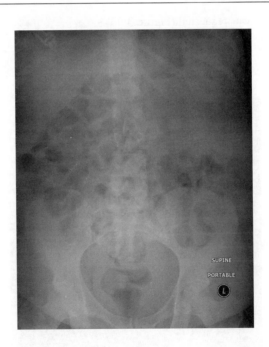

206. A supine abdominal projection was requested (Figure 3-72).

_____

_____

Figure 3-73

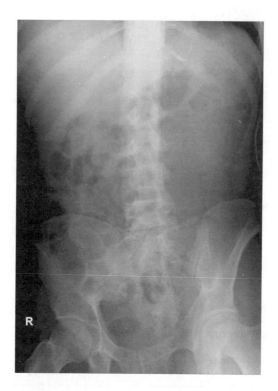

207. A supine abdominal projection was requested (Figure 3-73).

_____

_____

Figure 3-74

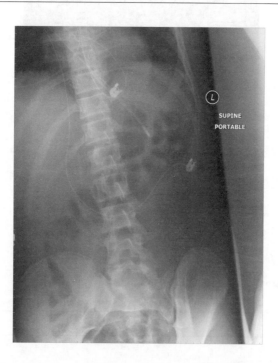

208. A supine abdominal projection was requested (Figure 3-74).

_____

_____

Figure 3-75

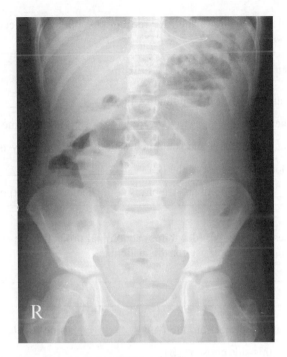

209. An upright abdominal projection was requested (Figure 3-75).

_____

_____

AP Projection (Left Lateral Decubitus Position)

210. Identify the labeled anatomy in Figure 3-76.

Figure 3-76

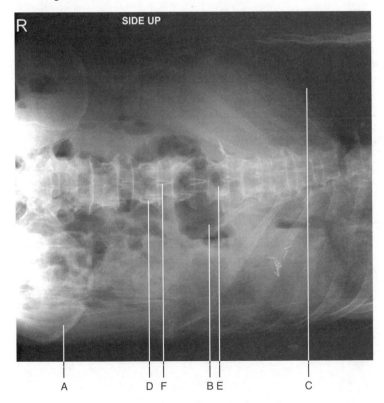

A. _____

B. _____

C. _____

D. _____

E. _____

F. _____

101

211. Complete the statements below referring to adult AP (decubitus) abdomen projection analysis guidelines.

> **AP (Decubitus) Abdomen Projection Analysis Guidelines**
>
> - Spinous processes are aligned with the midline of the (A) _____, and the distance from the pedicles to the (B) _____ is the same on both sides. The sacrum is centered within the inlet of the pelvis and is aligned with the pubis symphysis.
> - Diaphragm domes are located superior to the (C) _____ posterior ribs.
> - (D) _____ lumbar vertebra is at the center of the exposure field.

212. A patient's requisition requests that an AP (decubitus) abdominal projection be taken to rule out ascites. Describe how to determine the technique factors to use for this patient.

_____

_____

213. For an AP (decubitus) abdominal projection, the (A) _____ side of the patient is positioned against the imaging table or cart. Why is this side chosen? (B) _____

_____

214. Placing a pillow between the patient's knees for an AP (decubitus) abdominal projection will prevent

_____

215. To obtain optimal intraperitoneal air demonstration, the patient should remain in the decubitus position for

(A) _____ minutes before the AP (decubitus) projection is taken. Why is this time delay necessary?

(B) _____

216. Intraperitoneal air is most often found beneath the (A) _____ on an AP (decubitus) abdominal projection with proper positioning. Describe the shape of a patient's body that will result in the intraperitoneal air being demonstrated over the right iliac wing on a properly positioned AP (decubitus) abdominal projection.

(B) _____

217. What respiration is used for an AP (decubitus) abdominal projection?

_____

218. Which anatomic structures are included on an AP (decubitus) abdominal projection with accurate positioning?

_____

_____

For the following descriptions of AP (decubitus) abdominal projections with poor positioning, state how the patient would have been mispositioned or the CR misaligned for such a projection to be obtained.

219. The projection demonstrates a greater distance from the left lumbar vertebral pedicles to the spinous processes than the right pedicles to the spinous processes.

    _____

220. The projection demonstrates the upper abdominal region with equal distances from the vertebral pedicles to the spinous processes on each side, and the lower abdominal region demonstrates the sacrum and pubis symphysis without alignment. The sacrum is rotated toward the left pelvic inlet.

    _____

    _____

221. The projection demonstrates a clipped right diaphragmatic dome.

    _____

For the following AP (decubitus) abdominal projection with poor positioning, state which anatomic structures are misaligned and how the patient should be repositioned for an optimal projection to be obtained.

Figure 3-77

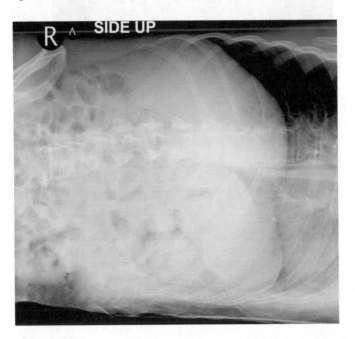

222. Figure 3-77:

    _____

    _____

Neonate and Infant: AP Projection

223. Identify the labeled anatomy in Figure 3-78.

Figure 3-78

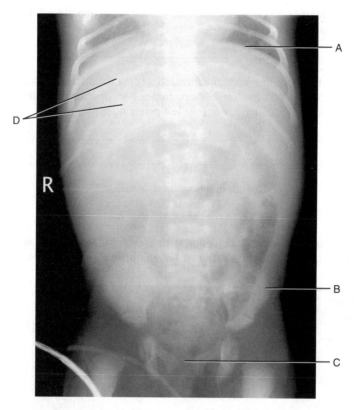

A. _____

B. _____

C. _____

D. _____

224. Complete the statements below referring to neonate and infant AP abdomen projection analysis guidelines.

AP Abdomen Projection Analysis Guidelines
■ Diaphragm domes are superior to the (A) _____ posterior rib.
■ (B) _____ vertebra is at the center of the exposure field.

225. To accurately center a neonatal and infant AP abdominal projection, the CR is centered to the (A) _____ plane at a level (B) _____ inches (C) _____ to the (D) _____.

For the following descriptions of neonatal or infant AP abdominal projections with poor positioning, state how the patient would have been mispositioned or the CR misaligned for such a projection to be obtained.

226. The diaphragm is not included on the projection.

_____

227. The patient's upper vertebral column is tilted toward the left side.

_____

228. The left inferior posterior ribs are longer than the posterior ribs on the right side.

_____

229. The right iliac wing is wider than the left wing.

_____

230. The diaphragm is at the level of the ninth posterior rib.

_____

For the following AP neonatal or infant abdominal projections with poor positioning, state which anatomic structures are misaligned and how the patient should be repositioned for an optimal projection to be obtained.

Figure 3-79

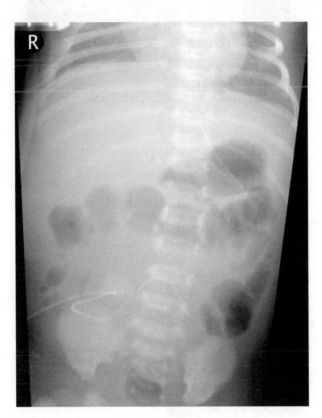

231. Figure 3-79:

_____

_____

Figure 3-80

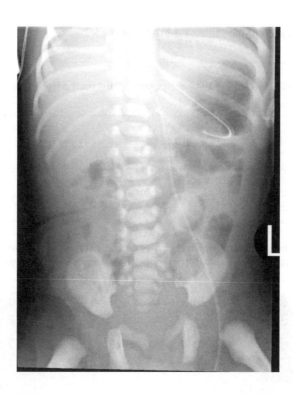

232. Figure 3-80:

_____

_____

Child: AP Projection

233. Identify the labeled anatomy in Figure 3-81.

Figure 3-81

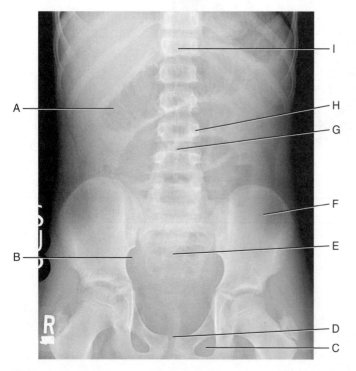

A. _____

B. _____

C. _____

D. _____

E. _____

F. _____

G. _____

H. _____

I. _____

106

For the following descriptions of child AP abdominal projections with poor positioning, state how the patient would have been mispositioned or the CR misaligned for such a projection to be obtained.

234. The distance from the right lumbar vertebral pedicles to the spinous processes is greater than the distance from the left pedicles to the spinous processes.

_____

_____

235. The left inferior posterior ribs are longer than the right, and the left iliac wing is wider than the right.

_____

_____

For the following AP child abdominal projections with poor positioning, state which anatomic structures are misaligned and how the patient should be repositioned for an optimal projection to be obtained.

Figure 3-82

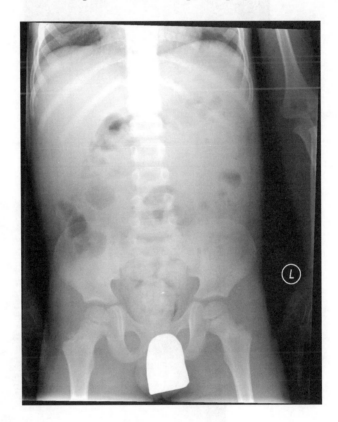

236. Figure 3-82, supine abdomen:

_____

_____

Figure 3-83

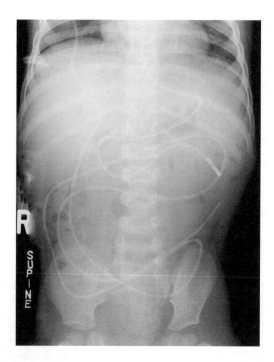

237. Figure 3-83, supine abdomen:

_____

_____

Figure 3-84

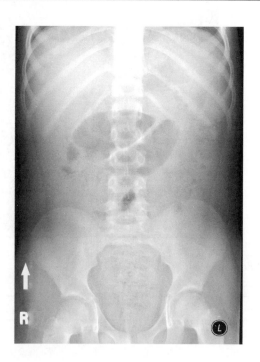

238. Figure 3-84, upright abdomen:

_____

_____

Neonate and Infant: AP Projection (Left Lateral Decubitus Position)

Figure 3-85

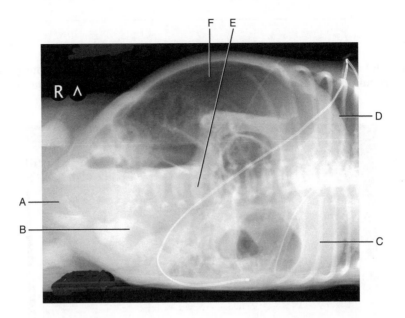

239. Identify the labeled anatomy in Figure 3-85.

A. _____

B. _____

C. _____

D. _____

E. _____

F. _____

240. Explain why the left side of the patient is placed adjacent to the bed or cart when the patient is positioned for neonatal or infant AP (decubitus) abdomen projections.

_____

_____

241. For a neonatal and infant AP (decubitus) abdominal projection, a horizontal CR is centered to the

(A) _____ plane at a level (B) _____ inches (C) _____ to the (D) _____.

For the following descriptions of neonatal or infant left AP (decubitus) abdominal projections with poor positioning, state how the patient would have been mispositioned or the CR misaligned for such a projection to be obtained.

242. The left iliac wing is narrower than the right iliac wing.

_____

_____

243. The diaphragm is not included on the projection.

_____

_____

244. The right posterior ribs are longer than the posterior ribs on the left side.

_____

_____

For the following neonatal or infant left AP (decubitus) abdominal projections with poor positioning, state which anatomic structures are misaligned and how the patient should be repositioned for an optimal projection to be obtained.

Figure 3-86

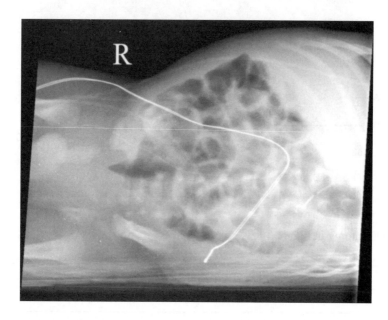

245. Figure 3-86:

_____

_____

Figure 3-87

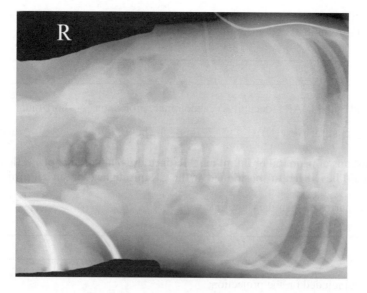

246. Figure 3-87:

_____

_____

Child: AP Projection (Left Lateral Decubitus Position)

Figure 3-88

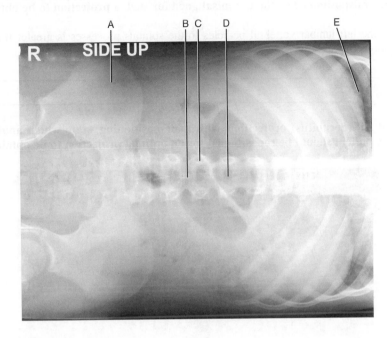

247. Identify the labeled anatomy in Figure 3-88.

A. _____

B. _____

C. _____

D. _____

E. _____

Figure 3-89

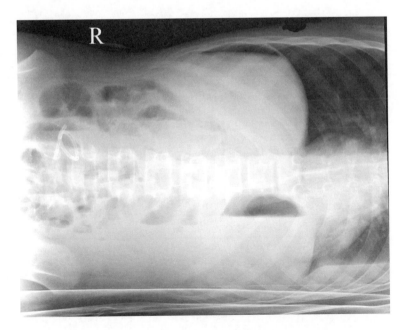

248. Identify the patient condition demonstrated on the projection in Figure 3-89.

Chapter **3 Image Analysis of the Chest and Abdomen**

For the following descriptions of child AP (decubitus) abdominal projections with poor positioning, state how the patient would have been mispositioned or the CR misaligned for such a projection to be obtained.

249. The distance from the left lumbar vertebral pedicles to the spinous processes is greater than that from the right pedicles to the spinous processes.

_____

_____

For the following child AP (decubitus) projections with poor positioning, state which anatomic structures are misaligned and how the patient should be repositioned for an optimal projection to be obtained.

Figure 3-90

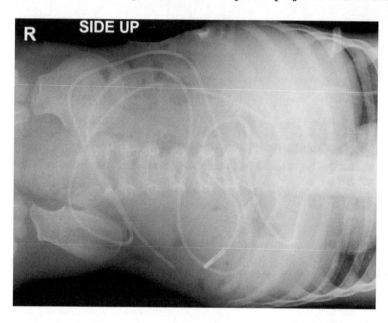

250. Figure 3-90:

_____

_____

Image Analysis of the Upper Extremity

STUDY QUESTIONS

1. Complete Figure 4-1.

Figure 4-1

Upper Extremity Technical Data				
Projection	kV	Grid	mAs	SID
Finger				
Thumb				
Hand				
Wrist				
Forearm				
Elbow				
Humerus				
Pediatric				

Finger: PA Projection

2. Identify the labeled anatomy in Figure 4-2.

Figure 4-2

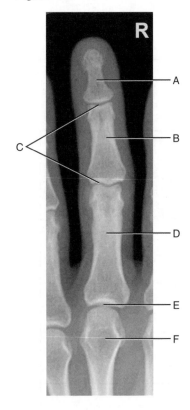

A. _____

B. _____

C. _____

D. _____

E. _____

F. _____

3. Complete the statements below referring to PA finger projection analysis guidelines.

PA Finger Projection Analysis Guidelines
■ Soft tissue width and the midshaft concavity are (A) _____ on both sides of phalanges.
■ IP and (B) _____ joints are demonstrated as open spaces, and the phalanges are seen without foreshortening.
■ The (C) _____ joint is at the center of the exposure field.
■ The entire finger and half of the (D) _____ are included within the collimated field.

4. To prevent finger rotation on a PA finger projection, the hand should be positioned _____ against the IR.

5. In which direction is the finger most frequently rotated when rotation occurs on a PA finger projection?

A. _____

Why?

B. _____

6. On a rotated PA projection, the side of the finger that is rolled (A) _____ (farther from/closer to) the IR will demonstrate the greatest phalangeal midshaft concavity and the (B) _____ soft tissue thickness.

7. Which of the finger MCs is the longest?

   _____

8. Which of the finger MCs is the shortest?

   _____

9. How is the patient positioned for a PA finger projection to prevent soft tissue overlap of adjacent fingers onto the affected finger?

   _____

10. To accomplish open joint spaces on a PA finger projection, the CR must be aligned (A) _____ (perpendicular/parallel) to the joint space, and the IR must be aligned (B) (perpendicular/parallel) _____ to the joint space.

11. If the finger is flexed for the PA projection, the joint spaces will be (A) _____, and the phalanges will be (B) _____.

12. On a patient whose finger is flexed, open IP joint spaces can be obtained by (A) _____ the hand and elevating the proximal MCs until the joint of interest is aligned (B) _____ to the IR.

13. Accurate CR centering is seen on a PA finger projection by centering a (A) _____ CR to the (B) _____ joint.

14. Included within the exposure field on a PA finger projection with accurate positioning are the (A) _____ and half of the (B) _____.

15. Accurate transverse collimation has been obtained when the collimated borders are _____.

For the following descriptions of PA finger projections with poor positioning, state how the patient would have been mispositioned for such a projection to be obtained.

16. The projection demonstrates unequal soft tissue width and midshaft concavity on each side of the phalanges. The side of the phalanges with the least amount of concavity is facing the longest finger MC.

   _____

17. The projection demonstrates closed IP and MCP joints, and the distal and middle phalanges are foreshortened.

   _____

For the following PA finger projections with poor positioning, state which anatomic structures are misaligned and how the patient should be repositioned for an optimal projection to be obtained.

Figure 4-3

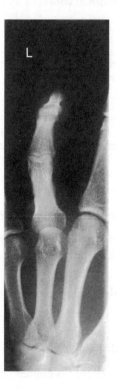

18. Figure 4-3: _____

_____

_____

Figure 4-4

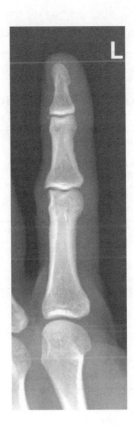

19. Figure 4-4: _____

_____

_____

_____

Finger: PA Oblique Projection

20. Identify the labeled anatomy in Figure 4-5.

Figure 4-5

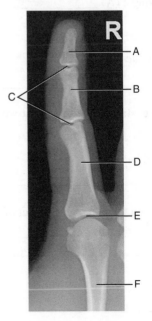

A. _____

B. _____

C. _____

D. _____

E. _____

F. _____

21. Complete the statements below referring to PA oblique finger projection analysis guidelines.

PA Oblique Finger Projection Analysis Guidelines
■ (A) _____ as much soft tissue width is demonstrated on one side of the phalanges as on the other side, and more (B) _____ is seen on one aspect of the phalangeal midshafts than the others.
■ IP and MCP joints are demonstrated as (C) _____ and the phalanges are not foreshortened.
■ The (D) _____ joint is at the center of the exposure field.

22. The affected finger is rotated _____ degrees from the PA projection for a PA oblique finger projection.

23. In which direction are the hand and finger rotated for a PA oblique projection when imaging the third through fifth fingers?

    A. _____

    For the second finger?

    B. _____

    Why is the second finger rotated differently?

    C. _____

24. To obtain open IP and MCP joint spaces, the finger needs to be fully (A) _____

    and positioned (B) _____ to the IR.

25. When imaging the third and fourth fingers, why is it often necessary to position a sponge beneath the distal phalanx?

    _____

26. Accurate CR centering on a PA oblique finger projection is accomplished by centering a (A) _____

    _____ CR to the (B) _____ joint.

27. Which anatomic structures are included on a PA oblique finger projection with accurate positioning?

    _____

For the following descriptions of PA oblique finger projections with poor positioning, state how the patient would have been mispositioned for such a projection to be obtained.

28. The soft tissue width and midshaft concavity are nearly equal on each side of the digit.

    _____

29. More than twice as much soft tissue width is present on one side of the phalanges as on the other. One aspect of the midshafts of the phalanges is concave, and the other aspect is slightly convex.

    _____

30. The projection demonstrates closed IP joint spaces, and the distal and middle phalanges are foreshortened.

    _____

For the following PA oblique finger projections with poor positioning, state which anatomic structures are misaligned and how the patient should be repositioned for an optimal projection to be obtained.

Figure 4-6

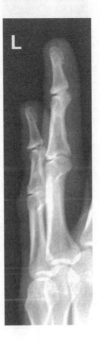

31. Figure 4-6, fourth digit: _____

_____

_____

Figure 4-7

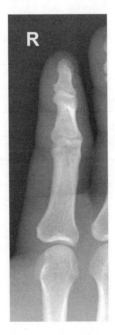

32. Figure 4-7, second digit: _____

_____

_____

Figure 4-8

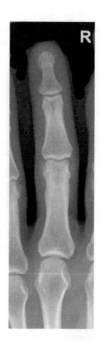

33. Figure 4-8, third digit: _____

_____

_____

Finger: Lateral Projection

34. Identify the labeled anatomy in Figure 4-9.

Figure 4-9

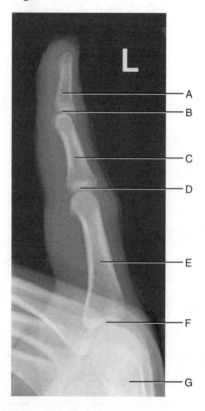

A. _____

B. _____

C. _____

D. _____

E. _____

F. _____

G. _____

35. Complete the statements below referring to lateral finger projection analysis guidelines.

Lateral Finger Projection Analysis Guidelines
■ (A) _____ surface of the middle and proximal phalanges demonstrate midshaft concavity, and the (B) _____ surfaces show slight convexity.
■ (C) _____ are demonstrated as open spaces, and the phalanges are not foreshortened.
■ (D) _____ is at the center of the exposure field.

36. For each of the following fingers, state how the hand is rotated (internally/externally) from the PA projection to place the finger in a lateral projection.

A. Second finger: _____

B. Third finger: _____

C. Fourth finger: _____

D. Fifth finger: _____

37. What determines how the hand is rotated for the previous question?

_____

38. How is the hand positioned for a lateral finger projection to prevent soft tissue overlap of the adjacent fingers onto the affected finger and to best demonstrate the affected finger's proximal phalanx?

_____

39. Which anatomic structures are included on a lateral finger projection with accurate positioning?

_____

40. Describe the positioning error that is demonstrated on the projection in Figure 4-10.

Figure 4-10

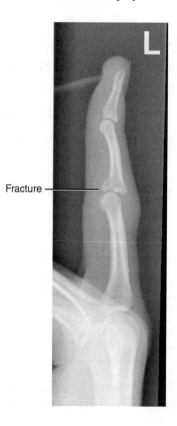

Fracture

_____

_____

For the following descriptions of lateral finger projections with poor positioning, state how the patient would have been mispositioned for such a projection to be obtained.

41. The proximal phalanges of the unaffected fingers overlap the proximal phalanx of the affected finger.

_____

42. Concavity is demonstrated on both sides of the middle and proximal phalangeal midshafts.

_____

43. The IP joint spaces are closed, and the phalanges are foreshortened.

_____

For the following lateral finger projections with poor positioning, state which anatomic structures are misaligned and how the patient should be repositioned for an optimal projection to be obtained.

Figure 4-11

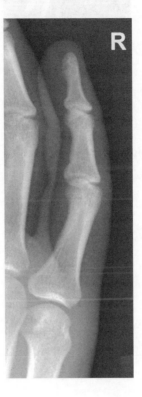

44. Figure 4-11: _____

_____

_____

Figure 4-12

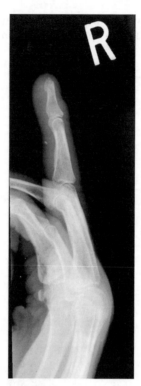

45. Figure 4-12: _____

_____

_____

Thumb: AP Projection

46. Identify the labeled anatomy in Figure 4-13.

Figure 4-13

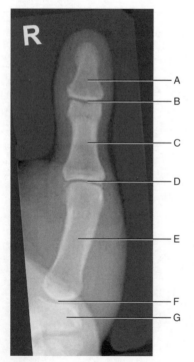

A. _____

B. _____

C. _____

D. _____

E. _____

F. _____

G. _____

47. Complete the statements below referring to AP thumb projection analysis guidelines.

AP Thumb Projection Analysis Guidelines
■ (A) _____ on both sides of the phalanges and MC midshafts is equal. Equal (B) _____ width on each side of the phalanges.
■ IP, MCP, and CM joints are demonstrated as (C) _____, and the phalanges are not foreshortened.
■ Superimposition of the (D) _____ soft tissue over the proximal first MC and the CM joint is minimal.
■ (E) _____ is at the center of the exposure field.

48. For the thumb to be positioned in an AP projection, the hand is (A) _____ (internally/externally) rotated, and the thumbnail is positioned (B) _____ against the IR.

49. When the thumb is rotated away from an AP projection, the amount of phalangeal midshaft concavity increases on the side positioned _____ (farther from/closer to) the IR.

50. To obtain open joint spaces on an AP thumb projection, the thumb is fully _____ and the CR is accurately aligned and centered to the thumb.

51. How is the hand positioned to prevent the medial palm soft tissue and possibly the fourth and fifth MCs from being superimposed over the proximal MC?

_____

52. Accurate CR centering on an AP thumb projection is accomplished by centering a (A) _____ CR to the (B) _____ joint.

53. List the anatomic structures that are included within the collimated field on an AP thumb projection with accurate positioning.

_____

For the following descriptions of AP thumb projections with poor positioning, state how the patient would have been mispositioned for such a projection to be obtained.

54. The soft tissue width and the concavity of the phalangeal and MC midshafts on each side are not equal. The side demonstrating the more concavity is facing toward the second through fifth digits, and the thumbnail is facing away from the second through fifth digits.

_____

55. The projection demonstrates a foreshortened distal phalanx and a closed IP joint space.

_____

56. The fifth MC and the medial palm soft tissue are superimposed over the proximal first MC and CM joints.

_____

For the following AP thumb projections with poor positioning, state which anatomic structures are misaligned and how the patient should be repositioned for an optimal projection to be obtained.

Figure 4-14

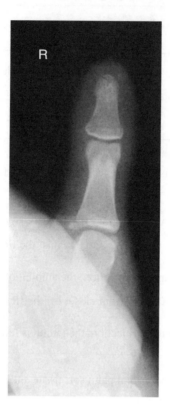

57. Figure 4-14: _____

_____

_____

Figure 4-15

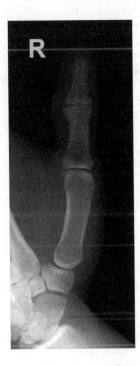

58. Figure 4-15: _____

_____

_____

Thumb: Lateral Projections

59. Identify the labeled anatomy in Figure 4-16.

Figure 4-16

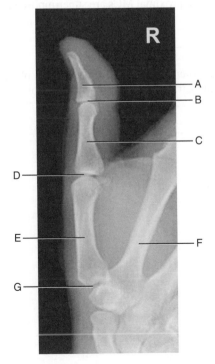

A. _____

B. _____

C. _____

D. _____

E. _____

F. _____

G. _____

60. Complete the statements below referring to lateral thumb projection analysis guidelines.

Lateral Thumb Projection Analysis Guidelines

- (A) _____ aspect of the proximal phalanx and MC demonstrates midshaft concavity, and the (B) _____ aspect of the proximal phalanx and MC demonstrates slight convexity.

- The IP, MCP, and CM joints are demonstrated as (C) _____, and the phalanges are not foreshortened.

- The proximal first MC is only slightly superimposed by the proximal (D) _____ MC.

- (E) _____ is at the center of the exposure field.

---

61. To obtain a lateral projection of the thumb, rest the hand flat against the IR and then _____ it until the thumb rolls into a lateral projection.

62. Abducting the thumb will decrease the amount of _____ superimposition of the CM joint.

63. Accurate CR centering on a lateral thumb projection is accomplished by centering a (A) _____ CR to the (B) _____ joint.

64. List the anatomic structures that are included within the collimated field on a lateral thumb projection with accurate positioning._____

For the following descriptions of lateral thumb projections with poor positioning, state how the patient would have been mispositioned for such a projection to be obtained.

65. The projection does not demonstrate a lateral projection. The second and third proximal MCs are superimposed over the first proximal MC.

_____

66. The projection does not demonstrate a lateral position. The anterior and posterior aspects of the proximal phalanx and MC midshafts demonstrate concavity. The first proximal MC is demonstrated without superimposition of the second and third proximal MCs.

_____

For the following lateral thumb projections with poor positioning, state which anatomic structures are misaligned and how the patient should be repositioned for an optimal projection to be obtained.

Figure 4-17

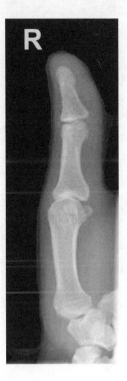

67. Figure 4-17: _____

_____

_____

Figure 4-18

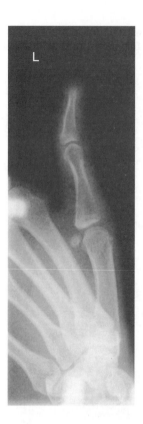

68. Figure 4-18: _____

_____

_____

Thumb: PA Oblique Projection

69. Identify the labeled anatomy in Figure 4-19.

Figure 4-19

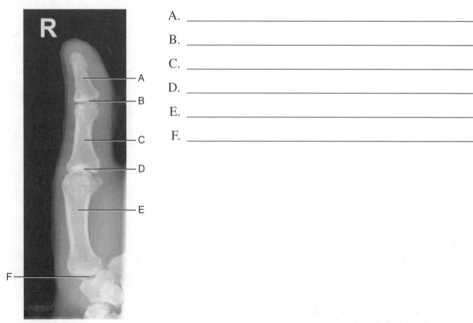

A. _____

B. _____

C. _____

D. _____

E. _____

F. _____

70. Complete the statements below referring to PA oblique thumb projection analysis guidelines.

PA Oblique Thumb Projection Analysis Guidelines
■ (A) _____ as much soft tissue, and more phalangeal and MC midshaft concavity are present on the side of the thumb next to the fingers than on the other side.
■ The IP, MCP, and CM joints are demonstrated as open spaces, and the (B) _____ are not foreshortened.
■ (C) _____ is at the center of the exposure field.

71. The affected thumb is rotated _____ degrees for accurate positioning for a PA oblique thumb projection.

72. The thumb is placed in a PA oblique projection when the hand is (A) _____, and the palm surface is placed

    (B) _____ against the IR.

73. Which anatomic structures are included on a PA oblique thumb projection with accurate positioning?

    _____

For the following description of a PA oblique thumb projection with poor positioning, state how the patient would have been mispositioned for such a projection to be obtained.

74. The midshafts of the proximal phalanx and MC demonstrate slight convexity on the posterior surfaces and concavity on the anterior surfaces.

    _____

For the following PA oblique thumb projections with poor positioning, state which anatomic structures are misaligned and how the patient should be repositioned for an optimal projection to be obtained.

Figure 4-20

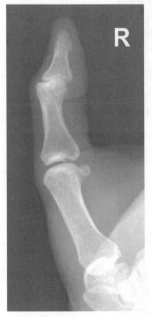

75. Figure 4-20: _____

    _____

    _____

Figure 4-21

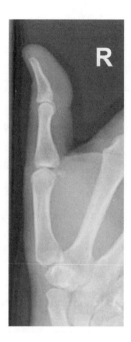

76. Figure 4-21: _____

_____

_____

Hand: PA Projection

77. Identify the labeled anatomy in Figure 4-22.

Figure 4-22

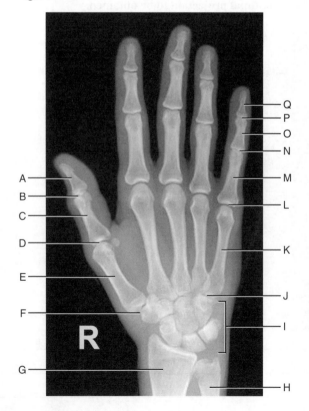

A. _____

B. _____

C. _____

D. _____

E. _____

F. _____

G. _____

H. _____

I. _____

J. _____

K. _____

L. _____

M. _____

N. _____

O. _____

P. _____

Q. _____

78. Complete the statements below referring to PA hand projection analysis guidelines.

PA Hand Projection Analysis Guidelines

■ Soft tissue outlines of the second through fifth phalanges are uniform, the distance between the
(A) _____ is equal, and the same midshaft concavity is seen on both sides of the
(B) _____ and MCs of the second through fifth fingers.

■ (C) _____, _____, and _____ joints are demonstrated as open spaces, and the phalanges are not foreshortened. The thumb demonstrates a 45-degree oblique projection.

■ (D) _____ is at the center of the exposure field.

---

79. To obtain a PA hand projection, (A) _____ the hand and place it (B) _____ against the IR.

80. What changes in the joint spaces, phalanges, and MCs would be expected on a PA hand projection if the hand is in a flexed position when it is taken?

_____

81. How will the position of the first digit change if the hand is flexed for a PA hand projection?

_____

82. Which anatomic structures are included on an accurately collimated PA hand projection?

_____

83. Why is a pediatric PA bone age hand image taken?

_____

84. Which hand is imaged for a pediatric PA bone age image?

_____

85. What are the reasons a child's pediatric skeletal and chronologic age may not correspond?

_____

For the following descriptions of PA hand projections with poor positioning, state how the patient would have been mispositioned for such a projection to be obtained.

86. The projection demonstrates superimposed third through fifth MC heads and unequal midshaft concavity of the phalanges and MCs.

_____

For the following PA hand projections with poor positioning, state which anatomic structures are misaligned and how the patient should be repositioned for an optimal projection to be obtained.

Figure 4-23

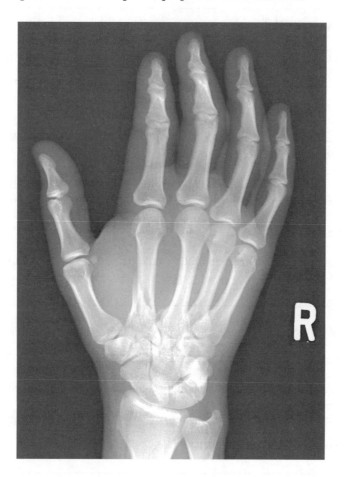

87. Figure 4-23: _____

_____

_____

88. The PA hand projection in Figure 4-23 demonstrates a proximal second MC fracture. If the patient could not move the hand from this position, how should the CR and IR be adjusted to obtain an optimal PA projection of this fractured MC?

_____

_____

Figure 4-24

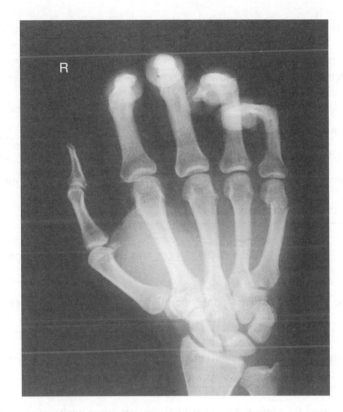

89. Figure 4-24: _____

_____

_____

Hand: PA Oblique Projection

90. Identify the labeled anatomy in Figure 4-25.

Figure 4-25

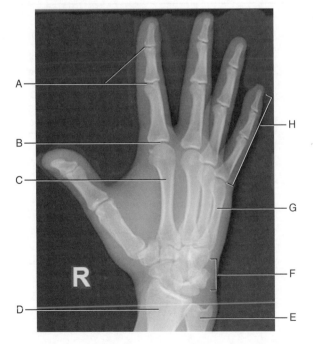

A. _____

B. _____

C. _____

D. _____

E. _____

F. _____

G. _____

H. _____

91. Complete the statements below referring to PA oblique hand projection analysis guidelines.

PA Oblique Hand Projection Analysis Guidelines

- Each of the second through fifth MC midshafts demonstrate more concavity on one side than on the other and have varying amounts of space between them. The (A) _____ MC heads are not superimposed, the (B) _____ MC heads are slightly superimposed, and a slight space is present between the (C) _____ MC midshafts.
- (D) _____ is at the center of the exposure field.

---

92. The hand is rotated (A) _____ degrees (B) _____ (internally/externally) from the PA projection for a PA oblique hand projection.

93. How must the fingers be positioned to demonstrate open IP and MCP joints on a PA oblique hand projection?

_____

94. Which anatomic structures are included on an accurately collimated PA oblique hand projection?

_____

For the following descriptions of PA oblique hand projections with poor positioning, state how the patient would have been mispositioned for such a projection to be obtained.

95. The MC heads are demonstrated without superimposition, and the spaces between the MC midshafts are nearly equal.

_____

96. The third through fifth MC midshafts are superimposed.

_____

For the following PA oblique hand projections with poor positioning, state which anatomic structures are misaligned and how the patient should be repositioned for an optimal projection to be obtained.

Figure 4-26

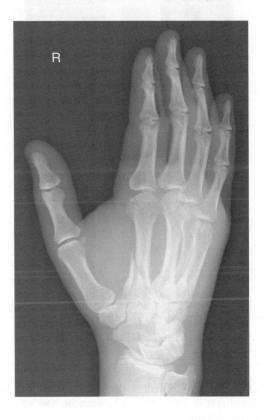

97. Figure 4-26: _____

_____

_____

98. The PA oblique hand projection in Figure 4-26 demonstrates a proximal second MC fracture. If the patient could not move the hand to adequately position it in a PA oblique projection, how should the CR and IR be adjusted for an optimal PA oblique projection to be obtained?

_____

_____

_____

Figure 4-27

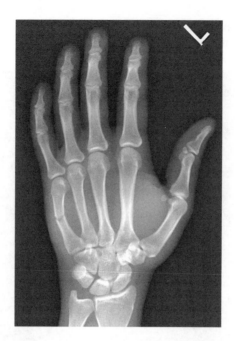

99. Figure 4-27: _____

_____

_____

100. The PA oblique hand projection in Figure 4-27 demonstrates a midshaft fifth MC fracture. If the patient could not move the hand to adequately position it in a PA oblique projection, how should the CR and IR be adjusted for an optimal PA oblique projection to be obtained?

_____

_____

_____

Hand: Lateral "Fan" Projection (Lateromedial)

101. Identify the labeled anatomy in Figure 4-28.

Figure 4-28

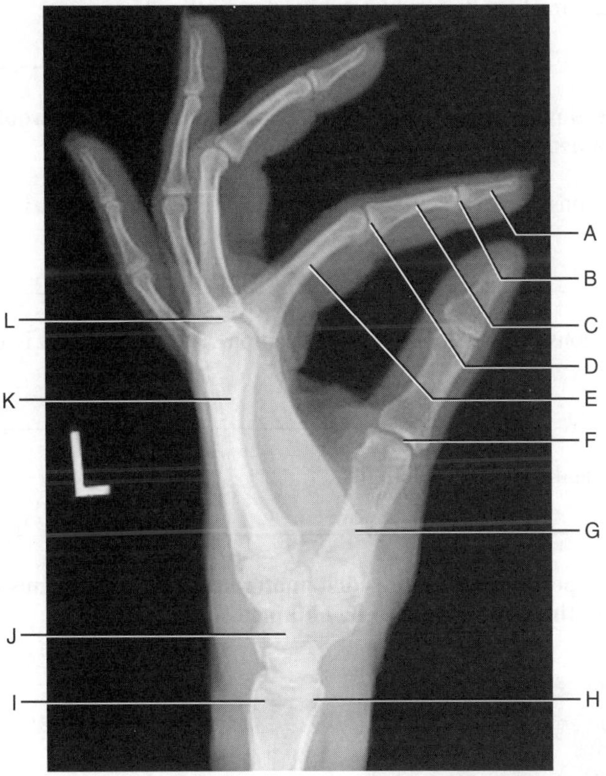

A. _____

B. _____

C. _____

D. _____

E. _____

F. _____

G. _____

H. _____

I. _____

J. _____

K. _____

L. _____

102. Complete the statements below referring to lateral hand projection analysis guidelines.

Lateral Hand Projection Analysis Guidelines

■ The second through (A) _____ digits are separated, demonstrating little superimposition of the bony or soft tissue structures.

■ The second through (B) _____ MCs are superimposed.

■ (C) _____ are at the center of the exposure field.

---

103. Why is it difficult to demonstrate the phalanges and MCs simultaneously on a fan lateral hand projection?

_____

104. For a fan lateral hand projection, the digits are most effectively fanned by drawing the second and third fingers (A) _____ (anteriorly/posteriorly) and the fourth and fifth fingers (B) _____ (anteriorly/posteriorly).

105. In what projection or position will the first digit be placed for accurate positioning for a lateral hand projection?

_____

106. How should the thumb be positioned to obtain open joint spaces and demonstrate the phalanges without foreshortening on a lateral hand projection?

_____

107. Which anatomic structures are included on an accurately collimated lateral hand projection?

_____

For the following descriptions of lateral hand projections with poor positioning, state how the patient would have been mispositioned for such a projection to be obtained.

108. The second through fifth MC midshafts are demonstrated without superimposition. The shortest MC is demonstrated anterior to the other MCs.

_____

109. The second through fifth MC midshafts are demonstrated without superimposition. The longest MC is demonstrated anterior to the other MCs.

_____

110. The projection demonstrates superimposed MCs and superimposed digits.

_____

For the following lateral hand projections with poor positioning, state which anatomic structures are misaligned and how the patient should be repositioned for an optimal projection to be obtained.

Figure 4-29

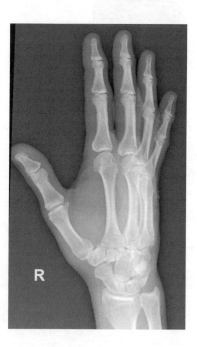

111. Figure 4-29: _____

_____

_____

Figure 4-30

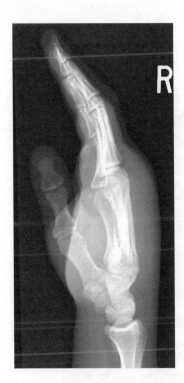

112. Figure 4-30: _____

_____

_____

Figure 4-31

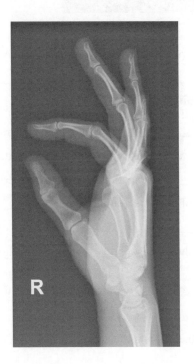

113. Figure 4-31: _____

_____

_____

Wrist: PA Projection

114. Identify the labeled anatomy in Figure 4-32.

Figure 4-32

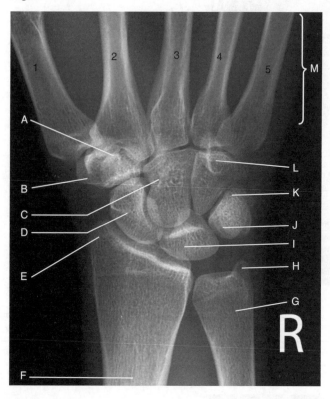

A. _____

B. _____

C. _____

D. _____

E. _____

F. _____

G. _____

H. _____

I. _____

J. _____

K. _____

L. _____

M. _____

115. Complete the statements below referring to PA wrist projection analysis guidelines.

PA Wrist Projection Analysis Guidelines
■ (A) _____ fat stripe is demonstrated.
■ Radial and ulnar styloids are at the extreme lateral and medial edges, respectively, of each bone. (B) _____ articulation is open, and superimposition of the MC bases is limited.
■ Anterior and posterior margins of the distal radius are not (C) _____.
■ (D) _____ CM joint spaces are open.
■ Long axes of the third MC and the (E) _____ are aligned with the long axis of the collimated field.
■ (F) _____ are at the center of the exposure field.

116. Describe the shape and location of the scaphoid fat stripe. _____

_____

117. Why is the visualization of the scaphoid fat stripe important on a PA wrist projection?

_____

118. To demonstrate the ulnar styloid in profile, the elbow is placed in a(n) (A) _____ projection, and the humerus is positioned (B) _____ with the IR.

119. The (A) _____ (anterior/posterior) margin of the distal radius is demonstrated distal to the (B) _____ (anterior/posterior) margin on a PA wrist projection with accurate positioning.

120. How is the forearm positioned for a PA wrist projection to obtain open radioscaphoid and radiolunate joint spaces?

_____

121. How is a patient with large muscular or thick proximal forearms positioned for a PA wrist projection to prevent demonstrating an excessive amount of the radial articular surface?

_____

122. How is the patient positioned for a PA wrist projection to obtain open second through fifth CM joint spaces?

_____

123. When the hand is placed on a flat surface, the wrist will be _____ (flexed/extended).

124. When the fifth MC and ulna are aligned with the long axis of the collimation field for a PA wrist projection, the distal scaphoid is (A) _____ (foreshortened/elongated), and the lunate moves (B) _____ (medially/laterally).

125. The lunate shifts _____ (medially/laterally) when the wrist is ulnar-deviated.

126. Accurate CR centering on a PA wrist projection is accomplished by centering a _____ CR to the wrist.

127. Which anatomic structures are included on an accurately collimated PA wrist projection?

_____

For the following descriptions of PA wrist projections with poor positioning, state how the patient would have been mispositioned for such a projection to be obtained.

128. The ulnar styloid is not demonstrated in profile.

_____

129. The laterally located carpal and MC joints are demonstrated as open spaces, and the medially located carpals and MCs are superimposed, closing the medially located carpal joints. The radioulnar joint is closed, and the radial styloid is not in profile.

_____

130. The laterally located carpals and MCs are superimposed, the pisiform and hamate hook are well demonstrated, and the radioulnar joint is closed.

_____

131. The posterior margin of the distal radius has been projected too far distal to the anterior margin.

_____

132. The scaphoid is foreshortened and the fourth and fifth CM joints are closed.

_____

133. The scaphoid is elongated and the second and third CM joints are closed.

_____

134. The scaphoid is foreshortened, the lunate is positioned mostly distal to the ulna, the third MC is not aligned with the long axis of the midforearm, and the CM joints are open.

_____

135. The scaphoid is elongated, the lunate is entirely positioned distal to the radius, and the third MC is not aligned with the long axis of the midforearm.

_____

For the following PA wrist projections with poor positioning, state which anatomic structures are misaligned and how the patient should be repositioned for an optimal projection to be obtained.

Figure 4-33

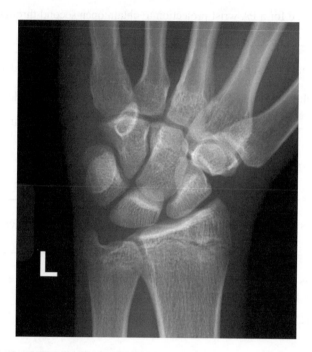

136. Figure 4-33: _____

_____

_____

Figure 4-34

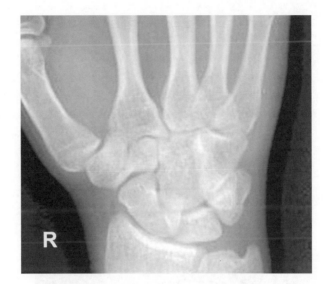

137. Figure 4-34: _____

_____

_____

Figure 4-35

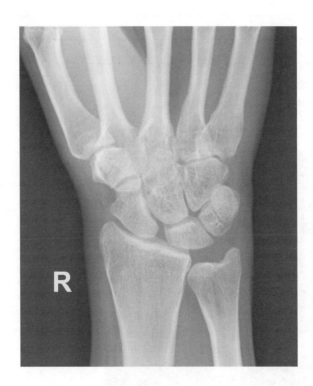

138. Figure 4-35: _____

_____

_____

Figure 4-36

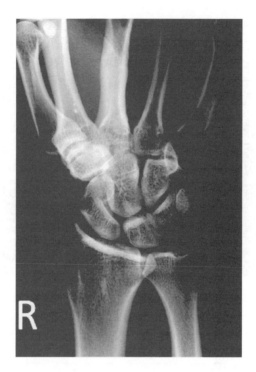

139. Figure 4-36: _____

_____

_____

Wrist: PA Oblique Projection

140. Identify the labeled anatomy in Figure 4-37.

Figure 4-37

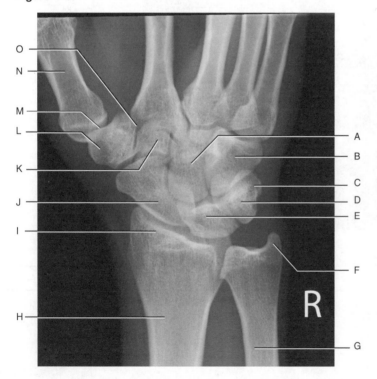

A. _____

B. _____

C. _____

D. _____

E. _____

F. _____

G. _____

H. _____

I. _____

J. _____

K. _____

L. _____

M. _____

N. _____

O. _____

141. Complete the statements below referring to PA oblique wrist projection analysis guidelines.

PA Oblique Wrist Projection Analysis Guidelines
■ (A) _____ and (B) _____ are demonstrated without superimposition, and the trapeziotrapezoidal joint space is open.
■ (C) _____ CM and scaphotrapezial joint spaces are demonstrated as open spaces.
■ (D) _____ is in profile at the far medial edge.
■ (E) _____ are at the center of the exposure field.

142. What routine degree of patient wrist rotation is required for a PA oblique wrist projection?

A. _____

As a routine, should the wrist be internally or externally rotated from a PA projection?

B. _____

143. For a PA projection of the wrist, the trapezoid and trapezium are superimposed. Which of these carpal bones is located anteriorly?

_____

144. The long axes of which two anatomic structures should be aligned when positioning the patient for a PA oblique wrist projection to ensure that no radial or ulnar deviation will result?

A. _____

B. _____

145. If the forearm is positioned parallel with the IR for a PA oblique wrist projection, how is the distal radius demonstrated on the resulting projection?

_____

146. On a PA oblique wrist projection with accurate positioning, the radioulnar joint space is closed. Which surface of the radius is superimposed over the ulna? _____ (anterior/posterior)

147. Accurate CR centering on a PA oblique wrist projection is accomplished by centering a _____ CR to the wrist.

148. Which anatomic structures are included on an accurately collimated PA oblique wrist projection?

_____

For the following descriptions of PA oblique wrist projections with poor positioning, state how the patient would have been mispositioned for such a projection to be obtained.

149. The trapezoid and trapezium demonstrate slight superimposition, obscuring the trapeziotrapezoidal joint space, and trapezoid-capitate superimposition is minimal.

_____

150. The third MC is pointing toward the lateral side of the wrist and the lunate is positioned laterally.

_____

151. The posterior margin of the distal radius superimposes less than one-fourth of the lunate.

_____

147

For the following PA oblique wrist projections with poor positioning, state which anatomic structures are misaligned and how the patient should be repositioned for an optimal projection to be obtained.

Figure 4-38

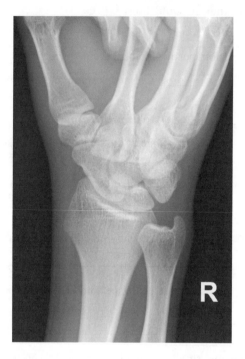

152. Figure 4-38: _____

_____

_____

Figure 4-39

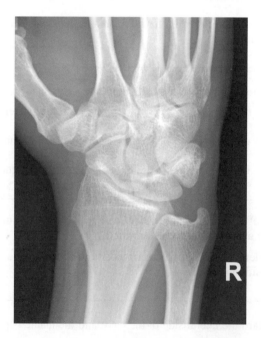

153. Figure 4-39: _____

_____

_____

Figure 4-40

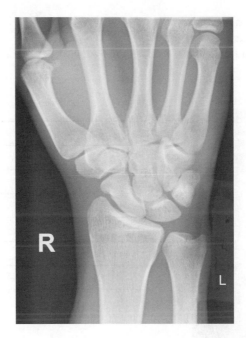

154. Figure 4-40: _____

_____

_____

Figure 4-41

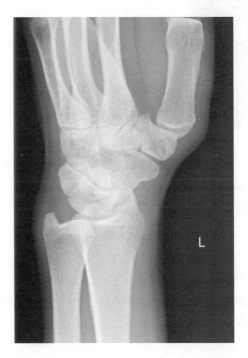

155. Figure 4-41: _____

_____

_____

Wrist: Lateral Projection (Lateromedial)

156. Identify the labeled anatomy in Figure 4-42.

Figure 4-42

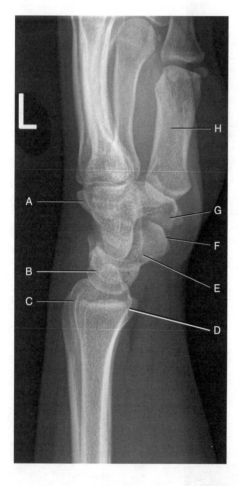

A. _____

B. _____

C. _____

D. _____

E. _____

F. _____

G. _____

H. _____

157. Complete the statements below referring to lateral wrist projection analysis guidelines.

Lateral Wrist Projection Analysis Guidelines
■ (A) _____ fat stripe is demonstrated.
■ (B) _____ aspects of the distal scaphoid and pisiform are aligned, and the distal radius and ulna are superimposed.
■ (C) _____ aspect of the distal scaphoid and pisiform are aligned.
■ The second through fifth MCs are placed at a (D) _____-degree angle with the anterior plane of the wrist.
■ The thumb is parallel with the (E) _____.
■ Ulnar styloid is demonstrated in profile (F) _____.
■ (G) _____ is demonstrated without superimposition of the first MC.

158. Describe the shape and location of the pronator fat stripe that is demonstrated on a lateral wrist projection with accurate positioning.

_____

_____

159. Why is the visualization of the pronator fat stripe on a lateral wrist projection of importance?

_____

160. Which side of the wrist is placed against the IR for a routine lateral wrist projection?

A. _____ (radial/ulnar)

What projection is this?

B. _____

In this projection, is the pisiform or distal scaphoid positioned closer to the IR?

C. _____

161. How are the hand and forearm aligned to prevent radial or ulnar deviation of the wrist for a lateral wrist projection?

_____

_____

162. Ulnar deviation of the wrist causes the distal scaphoid to be demonstrated (A) _____ (proximal/distal) to the pisiform, and radial deviation causes the distal scaphoid to be demonstrated (B) _____ (proximal/distal) to the pisiform on a lateral wrist projection.

163. If a patient with large muscular or thick proximal forearms is positioned without hanging the proximal forearm off the IR or imaging table, what type of wrist deviation will result? _____

164. For a lateral wrist projection, how is the patient positioned so that the wrist is in a neutral position without extension or flexion?

_____

165. How should one center the CR and collimate differently when a lateral wrist projection is ordered with the request that more than one-fourth of the distal forearm be included?

_____

166. For a lateral wrist projection, how are the humerus and elbow positioned to demonstrate the ulnar styloid in profile?

_____

167. For a lateral wrist projection, how are the humerus and elbow positioned to demonstrate the ulnar styloid projecting distal to the midline of the ulnar head?

_____

168. Which of the elbow and humeral positions described in the previous two questions demonstrates the ulna closer to the lunate on the resulting lateral wrist projection? _____

169. How is the patient positioned to prevent the first MC from being superimposed over the trapezium? _____

_____

170. Accurate CR centering on a lateral wrist projection is accomplished by centering a(n) _____ CR to the wrist.

171. Which anatomic structures are included on an accurately collimated lateral wrist projection? _____
_____

172. State whether the elbow was positioned in an AP or lateral projection for the wrist projections in Figure 4-43.

Figure 4-43

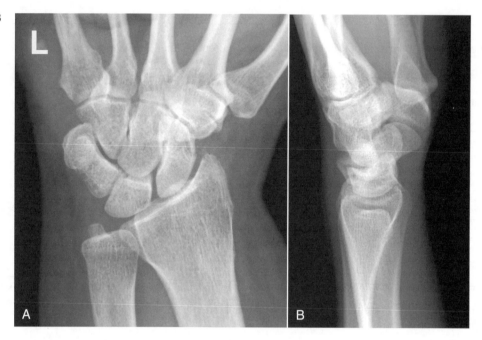

A. _____

B. _____

For the following descriptions of lateral wrist projections with poor positioning, state how the patient would have been mispositioned for such a projection to be obtained.

173. The pisiform is demonstrated anterior to the scaphoid, and the ulna is demonstrated anterior to the radius.
_____

174. The distal scaphoid is demonstrated distal to the pisiform.
_____

175. The ulnar styloid is projecting distal to the midline of the ulnar head. (In some facilities, this may not be considered poor positioning.)
_____

176. The first proximal MC is superimposed over the trapezium.
_____

For the following lateral wrist projections with poor positioning, identify the anatomic structures that are misaligned, state how the patient should be repositioned for an optimal projection to be obtained, and describe the position of the ulnar styloid.

Figure 4-44

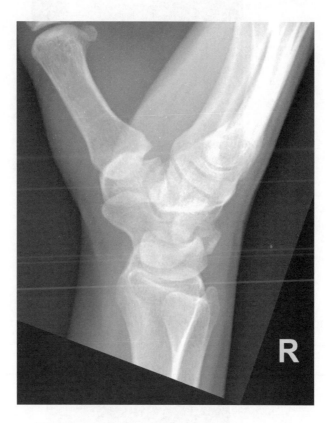

177. Figure 4-44: _____

_____

Ulnar styloid: _____ (profile/midline of ulnar head)

Figure 4-45

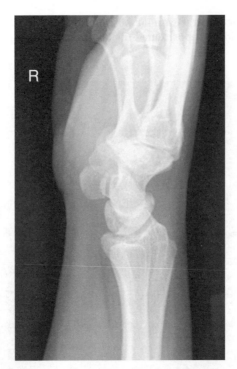

178. Figure 4-45: _____

_____

Ulnar styloid: _____ (profile/midline of ulnar head)

Figure 4-46

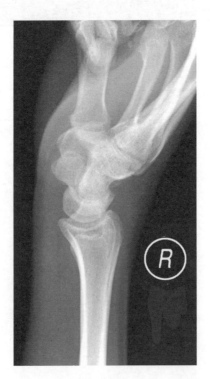

179. Figure 4-46: _____

_____

Ulnar styloid: _____ (profile/midline of ulnar head)

Figure 4-47

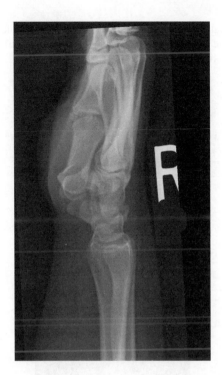

180. Figure 4-47: _____

_____

Ulnar styloid: _____ (profile/midline of ulnar head)

Figure 4-48

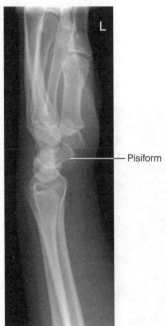

— Pisiform

181. Figure 4-48: _____

_____

Ulnar styloid: _____ (profile/midline of ulnar head)

182. (Figure 4-49) Because of the distal forearm fracture, the patient was unable to externally rotate the arm enough to obtain an accurate position for the wrist in a lateral projection. How should the CR have been adjusted from perpendicular to obtain accurate positioning?

Figure 4-49

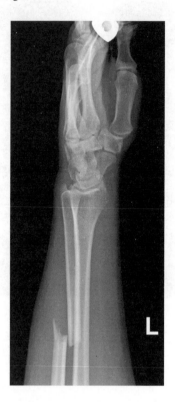

Wrist: Ulnar Deviation, PA Axial Projection (Scaphoid)

183. Identify the labeled anatomy in Figure 4-50.

Figure 4-50

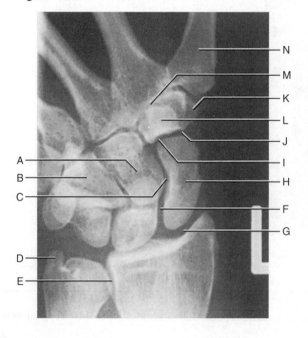

A. _____

B. _____

C. _____

D. _____

E. _____

F. _____

G. _____

H. _____

I. _____

J. _____

K. _____

L. _____

M. _____

N. _____

184. Complete the statements below referring to PA axial (scaphoid) wrist projection analysis guidelines.

PA Axial (Scaphoid) Wrist Projection Analysis Guidelines
■ (A) _____ and scaphotrapezoidal joint spaces are open.
■ Long axis of the (B) _____ and the radius are aligned.
■ Radioscaphoid, (C) _____, and scapholunate joints are open.
■ Ulnar styloid is in profile (D) _____.
■ (E) _____ is at the center of the exposure field.

185. Sufficient ulnar deviation of the wrist has been accomplished in the PA axial projection when the long axis of the (A) _____ and (B) _____ are aligned and the lunate is positioned distal to the (C) _____.

186. Why does ulnar deviation of the wrist increase the demonstration of the scaphoid?

_____

187. For a PA axial projection, how is the patient positioned to obtain open scaphocapitate and scapholunate joint spaces?

_____

188. If the wrist is adequately ulnar-deviated for the PA axial projection, how much and in which direction is the CR angled if a fracture of the scaphoid waist is suspected?_____

_____

189. What CR angulation is used if the patient is unable to adequately ulnar deviate for a PA axial wrist projection?

A. _____

Why is this adjustment needed?

B. _____

190. Where do most fractures occur on the scaphoid? _____

191. How is the CR angle adjusted for a PA axial wrist projection if a fracture of the distal scaphoid is suspected?

A. _____

If a proximal scaphoid fracture is suspected?

B. _____

192. If the CR is not aligned parallel with the fracture site for a PA axial wrist projection, will the fracture line be visible? _____ (Yes/No)

193. How is the patient positioned for a PA axial wrist projection to obtain an open radioscaphoid joint space?

_____

194. Which anatomic structures are included on a PA axial wrist projection with accurate positioning?

_____

_____

195. For the PA axial wrist projections in Figure 4-51, state whether a distal, waist, or proximal scaphoid fracture is demonstrated and the degree of CR angulation that should be used to best demonstrate each.

Figure 4-51

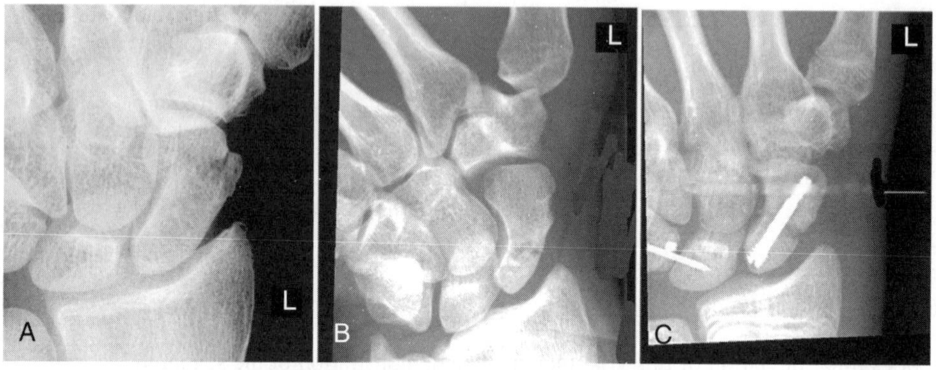

A. _____

B. _____

C. _____

For the following descriptions of PA axial wrist projections with poor positioning, state how the patient would have been mispositioned for such a projection to be obtained.

196. The scaphocapitate and scapholunate joints are closed, and the lunate is superimposed over a portion of the scaphoid.

_____

197. The scaphotrapezium, scaphotrapezoidal, and CM joint spaces are closed.

_____

For the following PA axial wrist projections with poor positioning, state which anatomic structures are misaligned and how the patient should be repositioned for an optimal projection to be obtained.

Figure 4-52

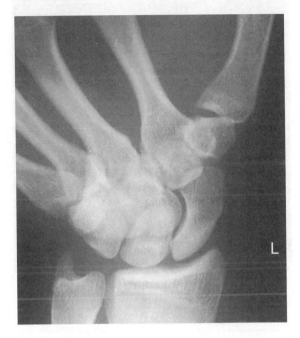

198. Figure 4-52: _____

_____

_____

_____

Figure 4-53

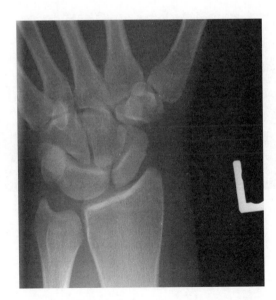

199. Figure 4-53: _____

_____

_____

_____

Chapter **4 Image Analysis of the Upper Extremity**

Figure 4-54

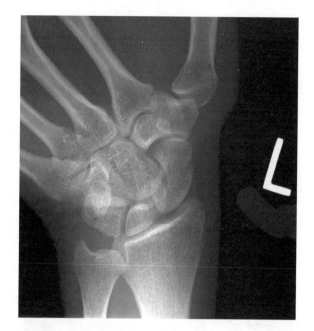

200. Figure 4-54: _____

_____

_____

_____

Wrist: Carpal Canal (Tunnel) (Tangential, Inferosuperior Projection)

201. Identify the labeled anatomy in Figure 4-55.

Figure 4-55

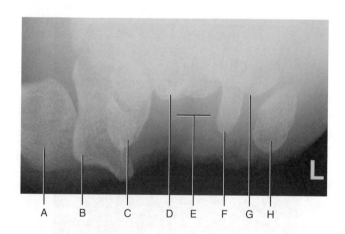

A. _____   E. _____

B. _____   F. _____

C. _____   G. _____

D. _____   H. _____

202. Complete the statements below referring to carpal canal wrist position analysis guidelines.

Carpal Canal Wrist Position Analysis Guidelines
■ (A) _____ is demonstrated without superimposition of the hamulus of the hamate.
■ (B) _____ canal is visualized in its entirety, and the carpal bones are demonstrated with only slight elongation.
■ (C) _____ is at the center of the exposure field.

203. The carpal canal projection is used to evaluate the carpal canal for (A) _____ and demonstrate

(B) _____ of the pisiform and hamulus of the hamate.

204. How is the patient positioned to demonstrate the pisiform without superimposition of the hamulus of the hamate

on the carpal canal projection?_____

205. To show the carpal canal and demonstrate the carpals with only slight elongation, the long axis of the MCs is

positioned close to (A) _____ with the wrist staying in contact with the IR, and the CR is angled

(B) _____ degrees proximally.

206. When imaging a patient who is unable to extend the wrist enough to place the MCs to within 15 degrees of vertical,

the CR angle needs to be (A) _____ (increased/decreased). If a 20-degree angle were required to bring
the CR parallel with the palmar surface in this situation, the angle needed for the carpal canal projection would be

(B) _____, and the resulting projection would show the carpals and carpal canal, although they will be

elongated because of the (C)_____.

**For the following descriptions of carpal canal wrist positions with poor positioning, state how the patient would
have been mispositioned for such a projection to be obtained.**

207. The pisiform is superimposed over the hamulus of the hamate.

_____

208. The carpal canal is not demonstrated in its entirety, and the carpal bones are foreshortened.

_____

209. The MC bases obscure the bases of the hamate's hamulus process, pisiform, and scaphoid.

_____

For the following carpal canal wrist positions with poor positioning, state which anatomic structures are misaligned and how the patient should be repositioned for an optimal projection to be obtained.

Figure 4-56

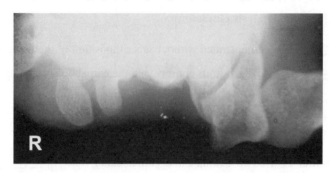

210. Figure 4-56: _____

_____

_____

_____

Figure 4-57

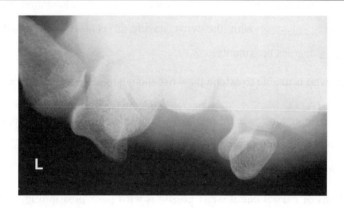

211. Figure 4-57: _____

_____

_____

_____

Figure 4-58

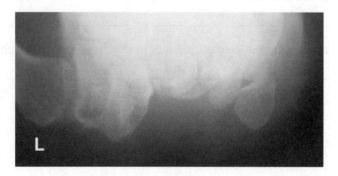

212. Figure 4-58: _____

_____

_____

_____

Forearm: AP Projection

213. Identify the labeled anatomy in Figure 4-59.

Figure 4-59

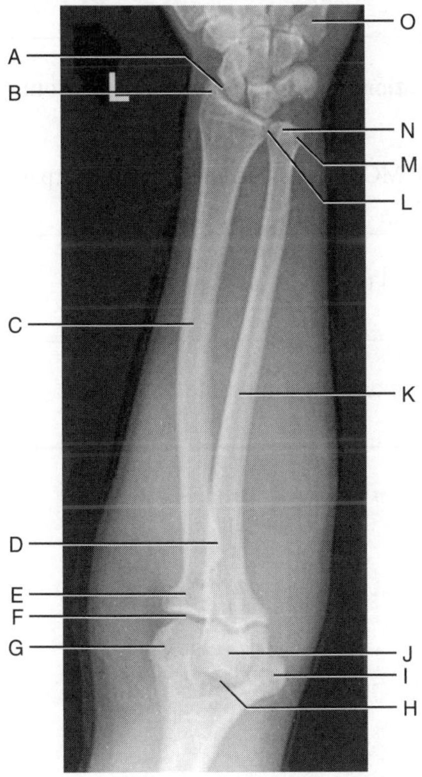

A. _____

B. _____

C. _____

D. _____

E. _____

F. _____

G. _____

H. _____

I. _____

J. _____

K. _____

L. _____

M. _____

N. _____

O. _____

214. How is the forearm positioned with respect to the x-ray tube to take advantage of the anode-heel effect?

_____

215. How can the location of the elbow joint be determined?

_____

216. On an AP forearm projection with accurate positioning, the (A) _____ is centered to the collimated field. This is accomplished by centering a (B) _____ CR to the (C) _____.

217. Which anatomic structures are included on an AP forearm projection with accurate positioning?

_____

218. An AP projection of the distal forearm has been obtained when the radial styloid is demonstrated in profile (A) _____ (medially/laterally), and superimposition of the radius and (B) _____ is minimal.

219. A patient from the emergency department is unable to position the wrist and elbow in an AP projection simultaneously for an AP forearm projection. How is this patient positioned for the projection?

_____

220. Why is the capitulum–radial joint partially or completely obscured on an AP forearm projection?

_____

221. On an AP forearm projection with accurate positioning, the radial tuberosity is demonstrated in profile, and the radius and ulna are visualized _____ with each other.

222. How is the patient positioned to place the radial tuberosity in profile on an AP forearm projection?

_____

For the following descriptions of AP forearm projections with poor positioning, state how the patient would have been mispositioned for such a projection to be obtained.

223. The distal forearm demonstrates superimposition of the first and second MC bases and laterally located carpal bones.

_____

224. The AP proximal forearm demonstrates the ulna without radial head and tuberosity superimposition.

_____

225. The radius is crossing over the ulna, and the radial tuberosity is not demonstrated in profile.

_____

226. Describe how the patient was positioned for the AP forearm projection in Figure 4-60.

Figure 4-60

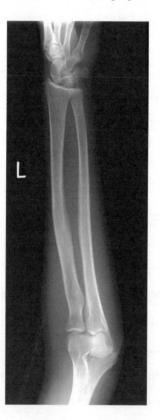

_____

_____

_____

227. The forearm projections in Figure 4-61 demonstrate a distal forearm fracture. Evaluate the accuracy of positioning in these two projections.

Figure 4-61

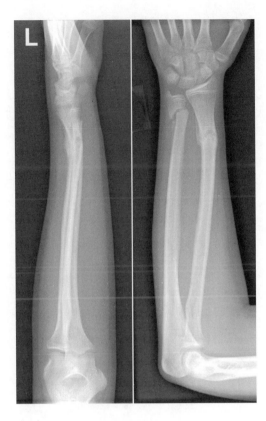

_____

_____

_____

_____

For the following AP forearm projection with poor positioning, state which anatomic structures are misaligned and how the patient should be repositioned for an optimal projection to be obtained.

Figure 4-62

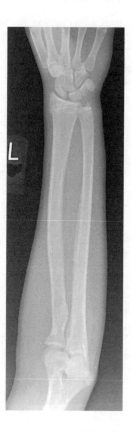

228. Figure 4-62: _____

_____

_____

_____

229. The AP forearm projection in Figure 4-63 demonstrates a midshaft radial fracture. If the patient could not move the forearm to adequately position it in an AP projection, how should the CR and IR be adjusted for an optimal AP forearm projection to be obtained?

Figure 4-63

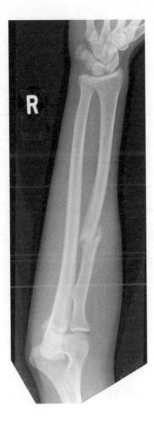

_____

_____

_____

_____

Forearm: Lateral Projection (Lateromedial)

230. Identify the labeled anatomy in Figure 4-64.

Figure 4-64

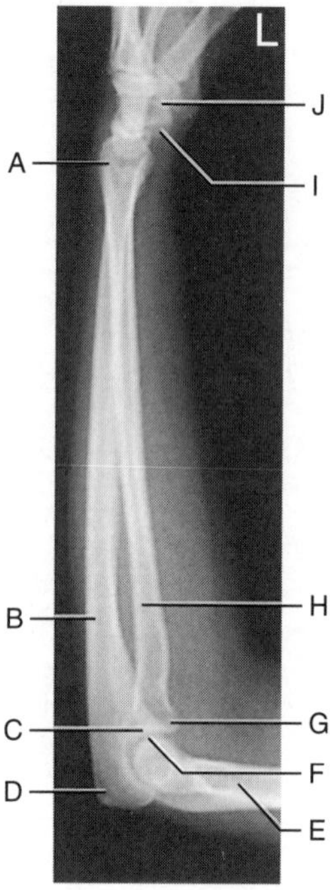

A. _____

B. _____

C. _____

D. _____

E. _____

F. _____

G. _____

H. _____

I. _____

J. _____

231. On a lateral forearm projection with accurate positioning, the _____ is centered within the collimated field.

_____

232. Which anatomic structures are included on an accurately collimated lateral forearm projection?

_____

233. On a lateral forearm projection with accurate positioning, the anterior aspect of the distal scaphoid and (A) _____ are aligned, and the distal radius and ulna are (B) _____.

234. On a lateral forearm projection with poor positioning, the ulna is demonstrated posterior to the radius. What will the distal scaphoid and pisiform relationship be?_____

235. Describe the placement of the ulnar styloid on a lateral forearm projection with accurate positioning.

A. _____

How must the patient be positioned to obtain this ulnar styloid positioning?

B. _____

236. Should the radial tuberosity be demonstrated in profile on a lateral forearm projection with accurate positioning?

A. _____ (Yes/No)

How is the patient positioned to obtain this positioning?

B. _____

168

237. In patients with average-size forearms, the elbow joint space is open on a lateral forearm projection. What two patient forearm shapes result in a closed elbow joint space?

_____

238. A lateral forearm projection with poor positioning demonstrates the capitulum distal to the distal surface of the medial trochlea. What is the radial head and coronoid relationship on this projection?

_____

239. A patient from the emergency department is unable to position the wrist and elbow in a lateral position simultaneously for a lateral forearm projection. The requisition states that the examination is being performed to rule out a proximal forearm fracture. How should the patient be positioned for this projection?

_____

_____

240. Evaluate the accuracy of the trauma lateral forearm projection in Figure 4-65. The patient could not position the distal and proximal forearm in a lateral projection at the same time.

Figure 4-65

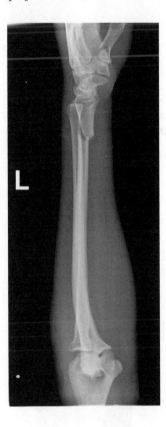

Chapter **4 Image Analysis of the Upper Extremity**

For the following descriptions of lateral forearm projections with poor positioning, state how the patient would have been mispositioned for such a projection to be obtained.

241. The pisiform is demonstrated anterior to the distal scaphoid, and the ulna is anterior to the radius. The proximal forearm demonstrates accurate positioning.

_____

242. The pisiform is visible posterior to the distal scaphoid, and the distal surface of the capitulum is demonstrated proximal to the distal surfaces of the medial trochlea.

_____

_____

243. The ulnar styloid is projecting distal to the midline of the ulnar head.

_____

244. The projection demonstrates the radial tuberosity in profile anteriorly.

_____

245. The radial head is demonstrated too far posterior on the coronoid process. The distal forearm demonstrates accurate positioning.

_____

For the following lateral forearm projection with poor positioning, state which anatomic structures are misaligned and how the patient should be repositioned for an optimal projection to be obtained.

Figure 4-66

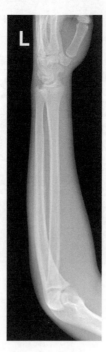

246. Figure 4-66: _____

_____

_____

_____

247. The lateral forearm projection in Figure 4-67 demonstrates a distal radial fracture. The patient's arm was externally rotated as far as possible. How should the CR and IR be adjusted for an optimal lateral forearm projection to be obtained?

Figure 4-67

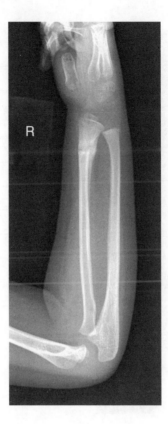

_____

_____

_____

_____

Elbow: AP Projection

248. Identify the labeled anatomy in Figure 4-68.

Figure 4-68

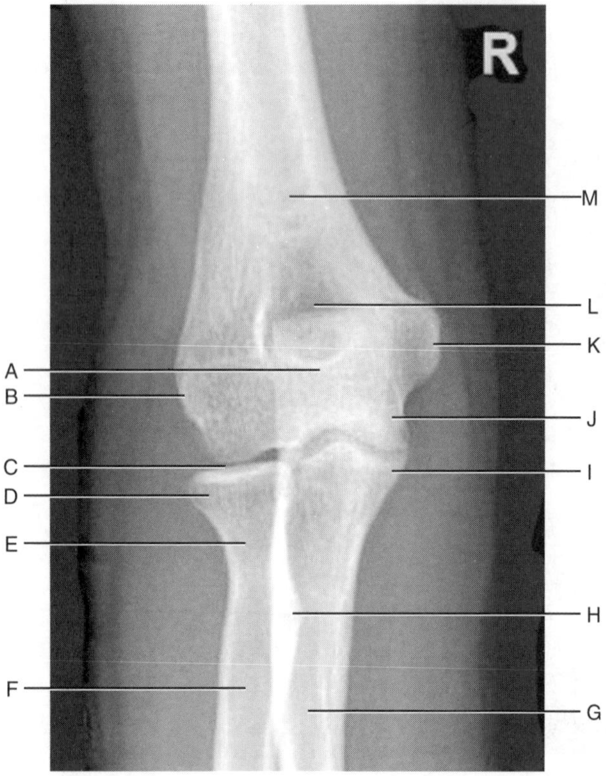

A. _____

B. _____

C. _____

D. _____

E. _____

F. _____

G. _____

H. _____

I. _____

J. _____

K. _____

L. _____

M. _____

249. Complete the statements below referring to AP elbow projection analysis guidelines.

AP Elbow Projection Analysis Guidelines

- Medial and lateral humeral epicondyles are demonstrated in (A) _____.

- One-eighth of the (B) _____ superimposes the proximal ulna.

- Radial tuberosity is in profile (C) _____, and the radius and ulna are parallel.

- The elbow joint is (D) _____.

- (E) _____ is at the center of the exposure field.

---

250. If the humeral epicondyles are accurately positioned for an AP elbow projection, what other structure can be manipulated to change the degree of radial tuberosity visualization?

_____

251. What two aspects of the positioning procedure need to be accurately set up to demonstrate the elbow joint space as an open space on an AP elbow projection?

A. _____

B. _____

252. A poorly positioned AP elbow projection demonstrates a closed elbow joint space. How can one determine if this closure was a result of poor CR placement or elbow flexion?_____

_____

_____

253. How is the patient positioned for an AP elbow projection if the elbow is unable to extend at least 30 degrees?

_____

254. Accurate CR centering on an AP elbow projection is accomplished by centering a (A) _____ CR (B) _____ (C) _____ to the medial epicondyle.

255. Which anatomic structures are included on an accurately collimated AP elbow projection?

_____

Figure 4-69

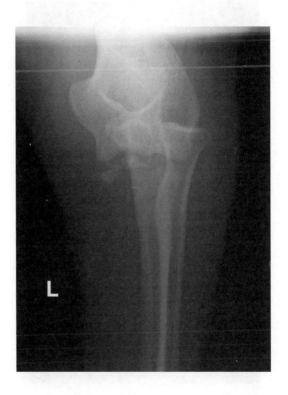

256. Which patient condition is demonstrated on the projection in Figure 4-69?

_____

_____

_____

For the following descriptions of AP elbow projections with poor positioning, state how the patient would have been mispositioned for such a projection to be obtained.

257. The radial head superimposes approximately half of the ulna.

_____

258. The projection demonstrates the radius crossing over the ulna, and the radial tuberosity is not shown in profile.

_____

259. The projection demonstrates a foreshortened proximal forearm and a closed capitulum–radial joint space.

_____

For the following AP elbow projections with poor positioning, state which anatomic structures are misaligned and how the patient should be repositioned for an optimal projection to be obtained.

Figure 4-70

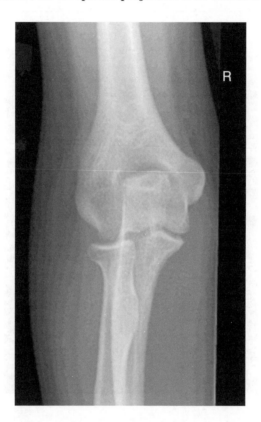

260. Figure 4-70: _____

_____

_____

_____

Figure 4-71

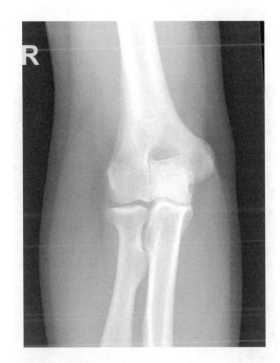

261. Figure 4-71: _____

_____

_____

Figure 4-72

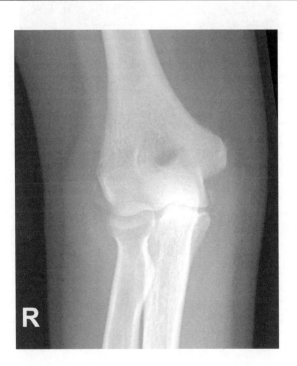

262. Figure 4-72: _____

_____

_____

_____

263. The AP projection in Figure 4-73 demonstrates a proximal radial fracture. If the patient could not move the arm to adequately position it for an AP projection, how should the CR and IR be adjusted for an optimal AP elbow projection to be obtained?

Figure 4-73

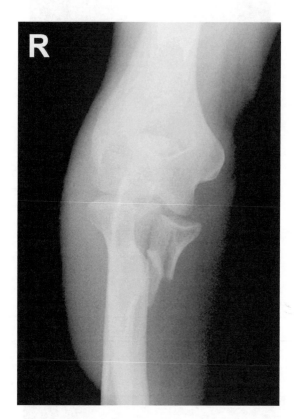

_____

_____

_____

264. The AP projection in Figure 4-74 demonstrates a distal forearm fracture that prevented the patient from internally rotating the arm the needed amount to obtain an accurate AP elbow projection. How should the CR and IR be adjusted to obtain an optimal projection?

Figure 4-74

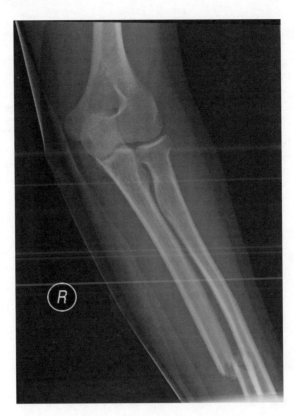

_____

_____

_____

_____

Elbow: AP Oblique Projections (Internal and External Rotation)

265. Identify the labeled anatomy in Figure 4-75.

Figure 4-75

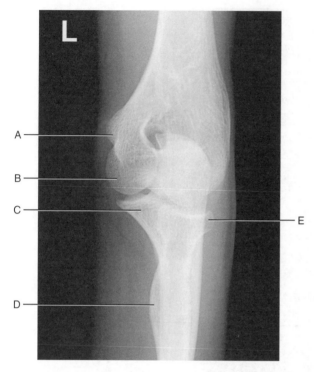

A. _____

B. _____

C. _____

D. _____

E. _____

266. Identify the labeled anatomy in Figure 4-76.

Figure 4-76

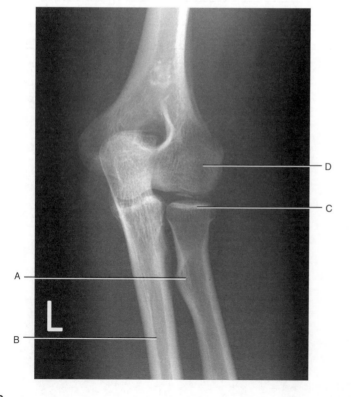

A. _____

B. _____

C. _____

D. _____

267. Complete the statements below referring to AP oblique elbow projection analysis guidelines.

AP Oblique Elbow Projection Analysis Guidelines

Medial oblique:

■ The coronoid process, trochlear notch, and (A) _____ are in profile.

■ (B) _____ joint space is open.

■ Three-fourths of the (C) _____ superimposes the ulna.

Lateral oblique:

■ The radial head and (D) _____ are in profile.

■ (E) _____ is demonstrated without radial head, neck, and tuberosity superimposition.

■ (F) _____ is at the center of the exposure field.

---

268. An AP oblique elbow projection with poor positioning demonstrates a closed capitulum–radial joint space. List two possible positioning problems that might have resulted in this projection.

   A. _____

   B. _____

269. State whether the forearm or humerus should be placed parallel with the IR to best demonstrate the anatomy listed below in a patient whose arm will not fully extend.

   A. Coronoid:_____

   B. Radial head:_____

   C. Medial trochlea:_____

   D. Capitulum:_____

   E. Capitulum–radial joint:_____

270. What is the degree of elbow rotation used for AP oblique projections?

   _____

271. Accurate CR centering on an AP oblique elbow projection is accomplished by centering a (A) _____

   CR to the elbow joint located at a level (B) _____ distal to the (C) _____

   _____.

272. Which anatomic structures are included on an AP oblique elbow projection with accurate positioning?

   _____

For the following descriptions of AP oblique elbow projections with poor positioning, state how the patient would have been mispositioned for such a projection to be obtained.

273. The externally rotated AP (lateral) oblique projection demonstrates a closed capitulum–radial joint space. The olecranon is positioned outside the olecranon fossa, and the radial articulating surface is demonstrated.

   _____

274. On the internally rotated AP (medial) oblique projection, the radial head is demonstrated lateral to the coronoid process, without complete superimposition of the ulna, and the proximal aspect of the olecranon is not demonstrated in profile.

_____

275. On the internally rotated AP (medial) oblique projection, more than three-fourths of the radial head superimposes the ulna.

_____

276. On the externally rotated AP (lateral) oblique projection, a portion of the radial head and tuberosity is superimposed over the ulna.

_____

277. On the externally rotated AP (lateral) oblique projection, the coronoid is superimposed over a portion of the radial neck, and the radial head and tuberosity are free of superimposition. The radial tuberosity is not demonstrated in profile.

_____

For the following AP oblique elbow projections with poor positioning, state which anatomic structures are misaligned and how the patient should be repositioned for an optimal projection to be obtained.

Figure 4-77

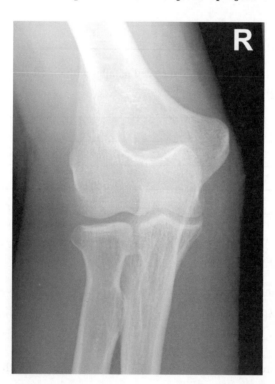

278. Figure 4-77, lateral oblique: _____

_____

_____

_____

Figure 4-78

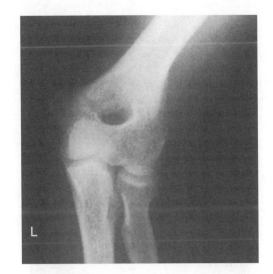

279. Figure 4-78, lateral oblique: _____

_____

_____

_____

Figure 4-79

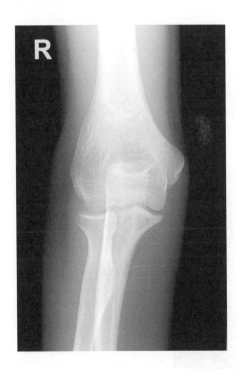

280. Figure 4-79, medial oblique: _____

_____

_____

_____

Figure 4-80

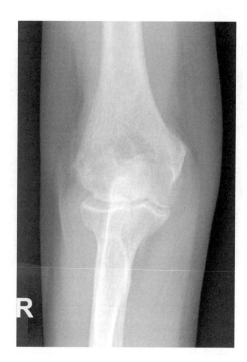

281. Figure 4-80, medial oblique: _____

_____

_____

_____

Elbow: Lateral Projection (Lateromedial)

282. Identify the labeled anatomy in Figure 4-81.

Figure 4-81

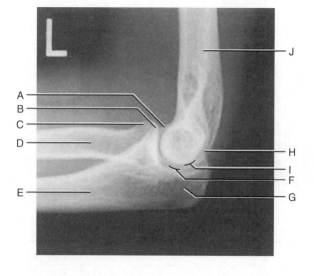

A. _____

B. _____

C. _____

D. _____

E. _____

F. _____

G. _____

H. _____

I. _____

J. _____

283. Complete the statements below referring to lateral elbow projection analysis guidelines.

> **Lateral Elbow Projection Analysis Guidelines**
>
> - The distal humerus demonstrates three concentric arcs, which are formed by the (A) _____, capitulum, and medial trochlea.
> - The elbow joint is open, and the proximal and (B) _____ surfaces of the radial head and the coronoid process are aligned.
> - The radial tuberosity is not demonstrated in (C) _____.
> - (D) _____ is at the center of the exposure field.

284. List the three soft tissue fat pads that may be demonstrated on a lateral elbow projection and describe their locations.

A. _____

B. _____

C. _____

Displacement of these pads may indicate what to the reviewer?

D. _____

285. Why is it important to flex the elbow 90 degrees for a lateral elbow projection?

_____

286. What three anatomic structures form the three concentric arcs on a lateral elbow projection with accurate positioning?

A. _____

B. _____

C. _____

Which of these arcs is the smallest?

D. _____

Which is the largest?

E. _____

How will improper alignment of these arcs affect the elbow joint space?

F. _____

287. A lateral elbow projection with poor positioning demonstrates the radial head positioned posterior on the coronoid process. How would the capitulum and medial trochlea be misaligned on this projection?

_____

288. The distal forearm was positioned too low for a lateral elbow projection. What will be the relationship between the radial head and coronoid and the capitulum and medial trochlea on the resulting projection?

_____

289. A lateral elbow projection with poor positioning demonstrates the capitulum too far posterior to the medial trochlea. How will the radial head and coronoid be aligned on this projection?

_____

290. The proximal humerus was positioned lower than the distal humerus on a lateral elbow projection. What will be the relationship between the radial head and coronoid and the capitulum and medial trochlea on the resulting projection?

_____

291. The position of the radial tuberosity on a lateral elbow projection is determined by the position of the hand and wrist. For the following positions, describe the location of the radial tuberosity.

A. Lateral hand and wrist: _____

B. Supinated hand and wrist: _____

C. Pronated hand and wrist: _____

Which of the radial tuberosity positions above is the desired position for an accurate lateral elbow projection?

D. _____

292. Accurate CR centering on a lateral elbow projection is accomplished by centering a (A) _____ CR to the elbow joint located (B) _____ inch(es) (C) _____ to the medial humeral epicondyle.

293. Which anatomic structures are included on a lateral elbow projection with accurate positioning?

_____

For the following descriptions of lateral elbow projections with poor positioning, state how the patient would have been mispositioned for such a projection to be obtained.

294. The olecranon is positioned within the olecranon fossa, and the posterior fat pad is demonstrated proximal to the olecranon process.

_____

295. The radial tuberosity is positioned in profile anteriorly.

_____

296. The radial head is positioned posterior on the coronoid process, and the distal surface of the capitulum is demonstrated distal to the distal surface of the medial trochlea.

_____

297. The radial head is positioned anterior on the coronoid process, and the distal surface of the capitulum is proximal to the distal surface of the medial trochlea.

_____

298. The radial head is distal to the coronoid process, and the capitulum appears anterior to the medial trochlea.

_____

299. The radial head is proximal to the coronoid process, and the capitulum appears posterior to the medial trochlea.

_____

For the following lateral elbow projections with poor positioning, state which anatomic structures are misaligned and how the patient should be repositioned for an optimal projection to be obtained.

Figure 4-82

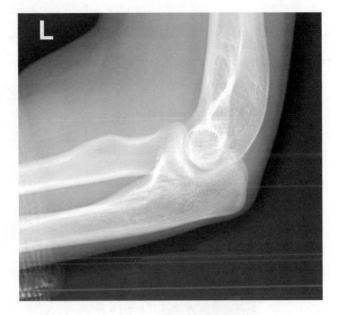

300. Figure 4-82: _____

_____

_____

_____

Figure 4-83

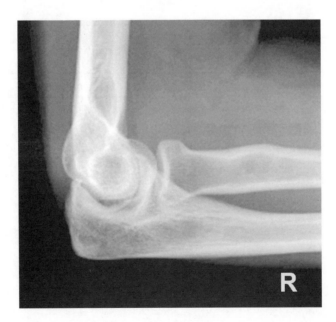

301. Figure 4-83: _____

_____

_____

_____

302. If the patient is unable to move the arm to adjust for the poor positioning demonstrated in Figure 4-83, how should the CR and IR be adjusted for an optimal lateral elbow projection to be obtained?

_____

_____

_____

Figure 4-84

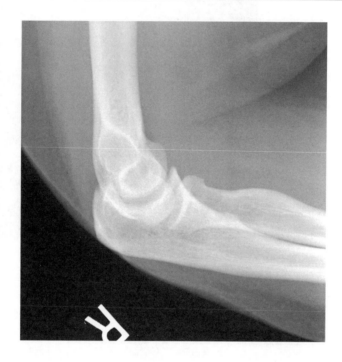

303. Figure 4-84: _____

_____

_____

_____

Figure 4-85

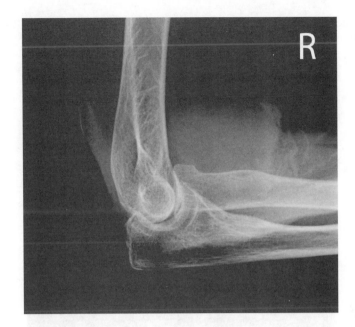

304. Figure 4-85: _____

_____

_____

_____

Figure 4-86

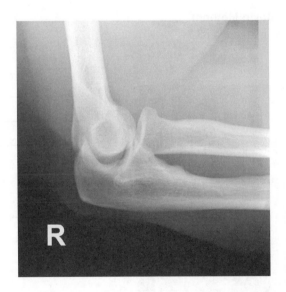

305. Figure 4-86: _____

_____

_____

_____

306. (Figure 4-87) The patient is unable to adjust positioning. How should the CR and IR be adjusted for an optimal lateral elbow projection to be obtained?

Figure 4-87

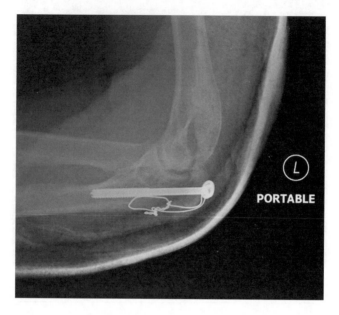

_____

_____

_____

Elbow: Axiolateral Projection (Coyle Method)

307. Identify the labeled anatomy in Figure 4-88.

Figure 4-88

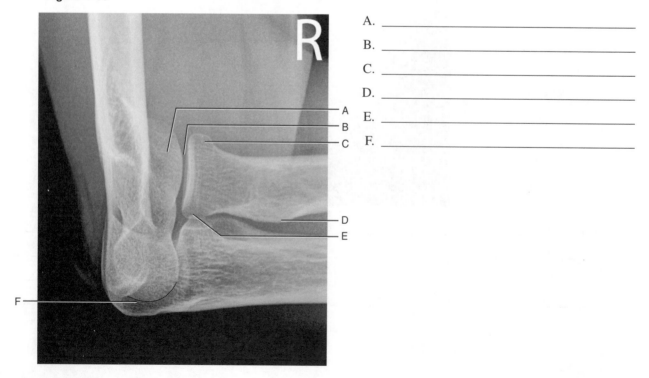

A. _____

B. _____

C. _____

D. _____

E. _____

F. _____

308. Complete the statements below referring to axiolateral elbow projection analysis guidelines.

Axiolateral Elbow Projection Analysis Guidelines
■ The capitulum is (A) _____ to the medial trochlea.
■ The radial head superimposes only the anterior tip of the (B)_____.
■ (C) _____ surfaces of the capitulum and medial trochlea are nearly aligned.
■ (D) _____ surfaces of the radial head and coronoid process are aligned.
■ (E) _____ is at the center of the exposure field.

309. What is the reason an axiolateral projection may be requested?

_____

310. In what position is the elbow placed to obtain the axiolateral projection of the elbow?

_____

311. The position of the distal forearm for an axiolateral projection affects the relationship of which anatomic elbow structures?

_____

_____

312. How can one determine from the projection if the forearm was elevated too high for the axiolateral elbow projection?

_____

_____

313. An axiolateral elbow projection with poor positioning demonstrates the radial head distal to the coronoid process. What is the relationship of the capitulum and medial trochlea on such a projection?

_____

314. To accurately separate the arcs of the distal humerus, an imaginary line connecting the humeral epicondyles is positioned (A) _____ to the IR, and a(n) (B)_____-degree CR angulation is directed (C) _____. Will this angle cause the radial head or coronoid to project farther anteriorly? (D) _____ Will this angle cause the medial trochlea or capitulum to project farther proximally? (E) _____

315. Which anatomic structure can be used to determine the portion of the radial head that is positioned in profile on an axiolateral elbow projection?

_____

Chapter **4 Image Analysis of the Upper Extremity**

316. For each of the following wrist projections, list the location of the radial tuberosity and the aspect of the radial head surface that are demonstrated in profile.

A. PA wrist: _____

B. Lateral wrist: _____

317. State which aspects of the radial head surface is demonstrated in profile on the projection in Figure 4-89.

Figure 4-89

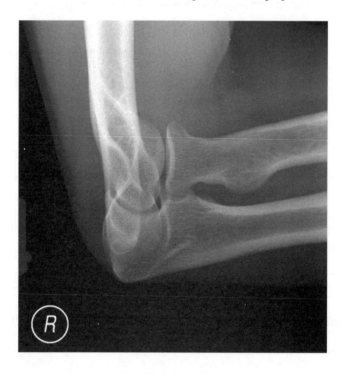

A. Anterior: _____

B. Posterior: _____

318. Accurate CR centering on an axiolateral elbow projection is accomplished by centering the CR to the:

_____

319. Which anatomic structures are included on an axiolateral elbow projection with accurate positioning?

_____

For the following descriptions of axiolateral elbow projections with poor positioning, state how the patient would have been mispositioned for such a projection to be obtained.

320. The capitulum–radial joint space is closed, the radial head is demonstrated proximal to the coronoid process, and the capitulum is demonstrated too far posterior to the medial trochlea.

_____

190

For the following axiolateral elbow projections with poor positioning, state which anatomic structures are misaligned and how the patient should be repositioned for an optimal projection to be obtained.

Figure 4-90

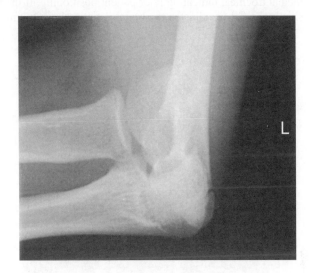

321. Figure 4-90: _____

_____

_____

_____

Figure 4-91

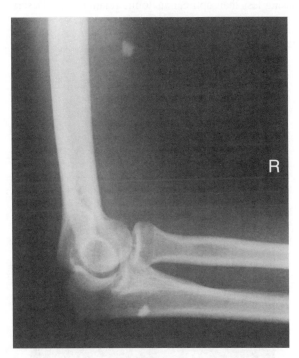

322. Figure 4-91: _____

_____

_____

_____

Chapter **4 Image Analysis of the Upper Extremity**

323. The axiolateral elbow projection in Figure 4-92 demonstrates a radial head fracture. Even though the projection was obtained with a 45-degree CR angle, the radial head is not anterior enough to the coronoid, nor is the capitulum proximal enough to the medial trochlea, indicating poor patient positioning. If the patient could not move the arm from this position, how should the CR be adjusted to obtain an optimal capitulum–radial head projection?

Figure 4-92

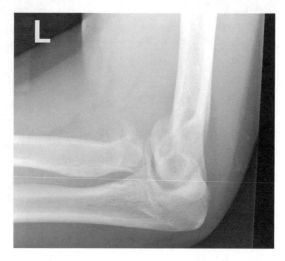

324. The patient was accurately positioned for the axiolateral elbow projection in Figure 4-93, but the CR was poorly aligned with the elbow, causing less than optimal anatomic relationships. Describe how the CR was aligned with the elbow to cause these results.

Figure 4-93

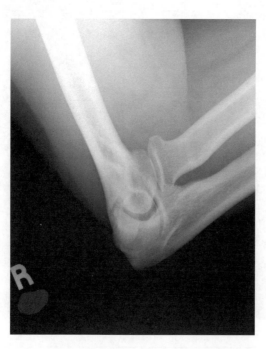

Humerus: AP Projection

325. Identify the labeled anatomy in Figure 4-94.

Figure 4-94

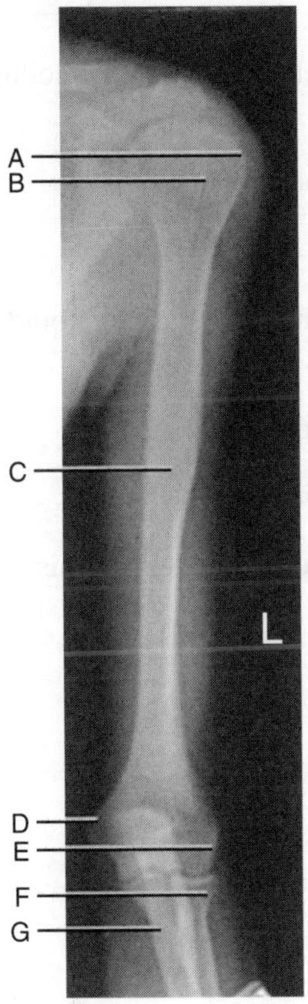

A. _____

B. _____

C. _____

D. _____

E. _____

F. _____

G. _____

326. An AP projection of the distal humerus has been obtained when _____ of the radial head superimposes the ulna.

327. On an AP proximal humeral projection with accurate positioning, the (A) _____ tubercle is demonstrated laterally in profile, the (B) _____ is demonstrated medially in profile, and the (C) _____ is visible approximately halfway between the greater tubercle and the humeral head.

328. If an AP humeral projection is ordered for a patient with a suspected proximal humeral fracture, why is it important not to rotate the arm externally?

A. _____

How can the ordered procedure still be performed without adjusting the arm position?

B. _____

329. An AP humeral projection is ordered for a patient with a humerus that is longer than 17 inches (43 cm). How should the arm be aligned with the IR to include the entire humerus on the same projection?

_____

330. Why is it necessary to have the IR and collimator light field extend beyond the shoulder and elbow joints when imaging the humerus in the AP projection?

_____

Chapter **4 Image Analysis of the Upper Extremity**

331. Describe how the shoulder and elbow joints can be located to ensure that the IR extends beyond each for an AP humeral projection.

    A. Shoulder:_____

    B. Elbow:_____

332. On an AP humeral projection with accurate positioning, the _____ is centered within the collimated field.

333. Which anatomic structures are included on an AP humeral projection with accurate positioning?

    _____

For the following descriptions of AP humeral projections with poor positioning, state how the patient would have been mispositioned for such a projection to be obtained.

334. The projection demonstrates the ulna without radial head and tuberosity superimposition.

    _____

For the following AP humeral projections with poor positioning, state which anatomic structures are misaligned and how the patient should be repositioned for an optimal projection to be obtained.

Figure 4-95

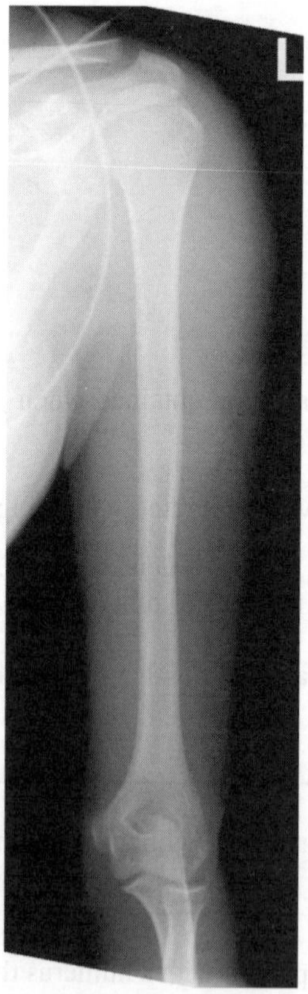

335. Figure 4-95: _____

    _____

    _____

    _____

Figure 4-96

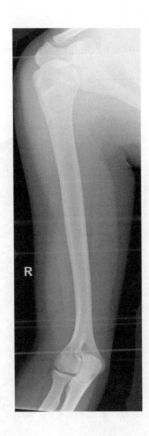

336. Figure 4-96: _____

_____

_____

_____

Humerus: Lateral Projection

337. Is the projection demonstrated in Figure 4-97 a mediolateral or lateromedial projection?

Figure 4-97

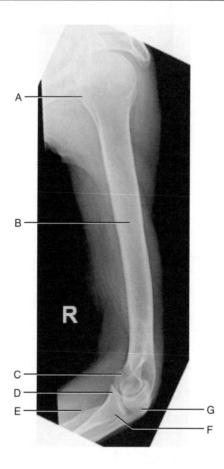

338. Identify the labeled anatomy in Figure 4-97.

A. _____

B. _____

C. _____

D. _____

E. _____

F. _____

G. _____

339. Identify the labeled anatomy in Figure 4-98.

Figure 4-98

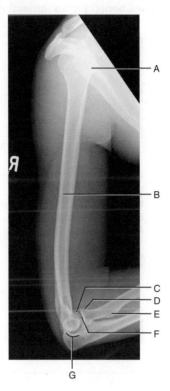

A. _____

B. _____

C. _____

D. _____

E. _____

F. _____

G. _____

340. A lateral humeral projection with accurate positioning demonstrates the (A) _____ tubercle in profile (B) _____ (medially/laterally).

341. When positioning the patient for a lateral humeral projection, the (A) _____ should be internally rotated until an imaginary line connecting the (B) _____ is positioned perpendicular to the IR.

342. List two alternative projections that can be used to position the humerus in the lateral projection in a patient with a suspected fractured proximal humerus.

A. _____

B. _____

343. On a lateral humeral projection with accurate positioning, the _____ is centered within the collimated field.

344. Which anatomic structures are included on a lateral humeral projection with accurate positioning?

_____

197

For the following lateral humeral projections with poor positioning, state which anatomic structures are misaligned and how the patient should be repositioned for an optimal projection to be obtained.

Figure 4-99

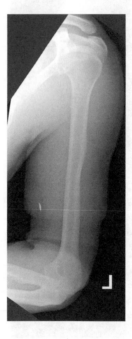

345. Figure 4-99: _____

_____

_____

_____

Figure 4-100

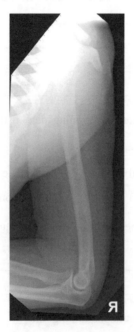

346. Figure 4-100: _____

_____

STUDY QUESTIONS

1. Routine shoulder projections are obtained using (A) _____ kV and (B) _____ SID.

2. When should a grid be used for the inferosuperior axial projection?

_____

Shoulder: AP Projection

3. Identify the labeled anatomy on Figure 5-1.

Figure 5-1

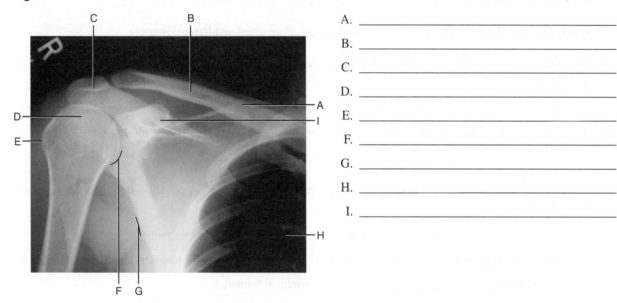

A. _____

B. _____

C. _____

D. _____

E. _____

F. _____

G. _____

H. _____

I. _____

4. Complete the statements below referring to AP shoulder projection analysis guidelines.

AP Shoulder Projection Analysis Guidelines

- The scapular body demonstrates minimal transverse foreshortening, and (A) _____ of the superior scapular body is visualized without thorax superimposition.

- The clavicle is demonstrated with minimal longitudinal foreshortening, with the medial clavicular end positioned adjacent to the (B) _____.

- The superior scapular angle is superimposed by the (C) _____.

- Neutral humerus: (D) _____ tubercle is partially seen in profile laterally and the humeral head is partially seen in profile (E) _____.

> - Externally rotated humerus: greater tubercle in profile (F) _____ and humeral head in profile (G) _____.
> - Internally rotated humerus: (H) _____ tubercle in profile medially and humeral head superimposed by the greater tubercle.

5. How is the patient positioned to prevent rotation on an AP shoulder projection?

   _____

6. What is the degree of scapular body obliquity on an AP shoulder projection?

   A. _____

   What portion of the scapula is situated anteriorly?

   B. _____

7. A nondislocated shoulder demonstrates slight superimposition of the humeral head and _____.

8. Which shoulder dislocation is the most common? _____ (anterior/posterior)

9. How is the patient positioned to demonstrate the scapular body without longitudinal foreshortening on an AP shoulder projection?

   _____

10. If the scapula is longitudinally foreshortened, the superior scapular angle is projected inferiorly or superiorly to the

    _____.

11. How can longitudinal scapular foreshortening be reduced when obtaining an AP shoulder projection on a patient with kyphosis?

    _____

12. The lateral humeral epicondyle is aligned with the (A) _____ tubercle, and the medial epicondyle is aligned with the (B) _____ of the proximal humerus.

13. State how the humeral epicondyles are positioned in reference to the IR to place the anatomic structures as described on the following AP shoulder projections.

    A. Greater tubercle is partially in profile laterally: _____

    B. Lesser tubercle is in profile medially: _____

    C. Greater tubercle is in profile laterally: _____

    D. Humeral head is in profile medially: _____

14. How is the patient's arm positioned for an AP shoulder projection if a shoulder dislocation or humeral fracture is suspected?

_____

15. Accurate CR centering on an AP shoulder projection is accomplished by centering a(n) (A) _____

CR 1 inch (2.5 cm) (B) _____ to the coracoid process.

16. Which anatomic structures are demonstrated within the exposure field on an AP shoulder projection with accurate collimation?

_____

For the following descriptions of AP shoulder projections with poor positioning, state how the patient would have been mispositioned for such a projection to be obtained.

17. The glenoid cavity is nearly in profile with only a small amount of the articulating surface demonstrated, the superolateral border of the scapula is superimposed by the thorax, and the medial clavicular end has been rolled away from the vertebral column.

_____

_____

18. The scapular body is drawn from beneath the thorax and is transversely foreshortened, the glenoid cavity is demonstrated on end, and the medial clavicular end is superimposed over the vertebral column.

_____

_____

19. The superior scapular angle is demonstrated superior to the clavicle, and the acromion process and humeral head demonstrate no superimposition.

_____

_____

20. A neutral shoulder projection demonstrates the greater tubercle in profile laterally and the humeral head in profile medially.

_____

_____

21. A neutral shoulder projection demonstrates the lesser tubercle in profile medially.

_____

_____

For the following AP shoulder projections with poor positioning, state which anatomic structures are misaligned and how the patient should be repositioned for an optimal projection to be obtained.

Figure 5-2

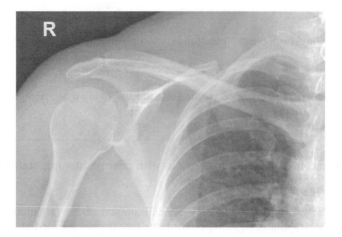

22. Figure 5-2: _____

_____

_____

Figure 5-3

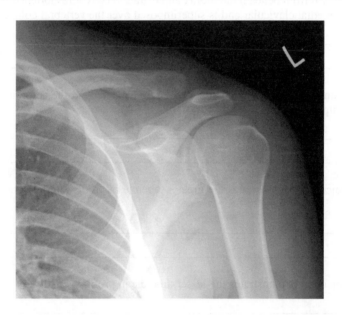

23. Figure 5-3: _____

_____

_____

Figure 5-4

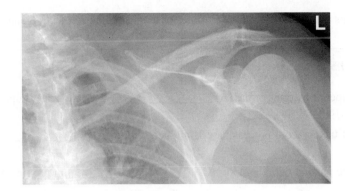

24. Figure 5-4: _____

_____

_____

Shoulder: Inferosuperior Axial Projection

25. Identify the labeled anatomy in Figure 5-5.

Figure 5-5

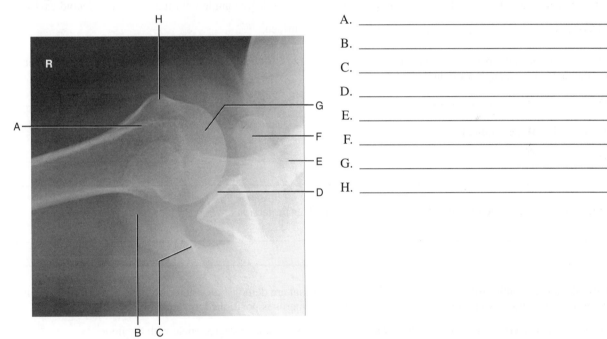

A. _____

B. _____

C. _____

D. _____

E. _____

F. _____

G. _____

H. _____

26. Complete the statements below referring to inferosuperior axial shoulder projection analysis guidelines.

Inferosuperior Axial Shoulder Projection Analysis Guidelines
■ The inferior and superior margins of the (A) _____ are nearly superimposed, demonstrating an open glenohumeral joint space.
■ The lateral edge of the coracoid process base is aligned with the (B) _____ glenoid cavity margin.
■ The epicondyles are parallel with the floor: (C) _____ in profile anteriorly.
■ The epicondyles are at a 45-degree angle with the floor: (D) _____ in partial profile anteriorly and the posterolateral aspect of the humeral head is in profile (E) _____.
■ The (F) _____ is at the center of the exposure field.

27. Humeral abduction of the arm is obtained by combined movements of the (A) _____ and

(B) _____.

28. On a patient who has no trouble abducting the humerus to a 90-degree angle with the body, the glenoid cavity is

placed at a _____ angle with the lateral body surface.

29. How should the angle between the lateral body surface and the CR be adjusted if the patient can abduct the humerus to only a 45-degree angle with the body?

A. _____

Why is this change required?

B. _____

_____

30. How is the IR positioned for an inferosuperior axial shoulder projection?

_____

_____

31. Describe the anatomic structures of the proximal humerus that are demonstrated anteriorly and posteriorly in profile on an inferosuperior axial shoulder projection when the humerus is positioned as stated below.

A. The arm is externally rotated until the humeral epicondyles are at a 45-degree angle with the floor.

_____

_____

B. The arm is externally rotated until the humeral epicondyles are perpendicular to the floor.

_____

_____

C. The arm is externally rotated until the humeral epicondyles are parallel with the floor.

_____

32. Accurate CR centering on an inferiorsuperior axial shoulder projection is accomplished by centering a (A) _____ CR to the midaxillary region at the same transverse level as the (B) _____.

33. Which anatomic structures are included on an inferosuperior axial shoulder projection with accurate positioning?

_____

34. For an inferosuperior axial shoulder, elevation of the shoulder on a sponge or washcloth prevents clipping of the _____ aspect of the humerus and shoulder.

35. Lateral neck flexion and turning the face away from the affected shoulder prevents clipping of the _____.

36. How were the humeral epicondyles positioned for the following inferosuperior axial shoulder projections?

Figure 5-6

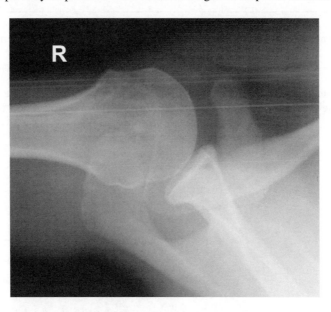

A. Figure 5-6: _____

Figure 5-7

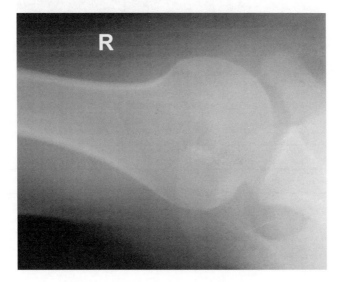

B. Figure 5-7: _____

205

For the following descriptions of inferosuperior axial shoulder projections with poor positioning, state how the patient would have been mispositioned or the CR aligned for such a projection to be obtained.

37. The glenohumeral joint space is obscured, and the inferior glenoid cavity is demonstrated lateral to the coracoid process base.

_____

38. The glenohumeral joint space is obscured, and the inferior glenoid cavity is demonstrated medial to the lateral edge of the coracoid process base.

_____

39. The greater tubercle is demonstrated in profile posteriorly.

_____

40. The acromion process, scapular spine, and posterior aspect of the proximal humerus were not included on the projection.

_____

For the following inferosuperior axial shoulder projections with poor positioning, state which anatomic structures are misaligned and how the patient should be repositioned for an optimal projection to be obtained.

Figure 5-8

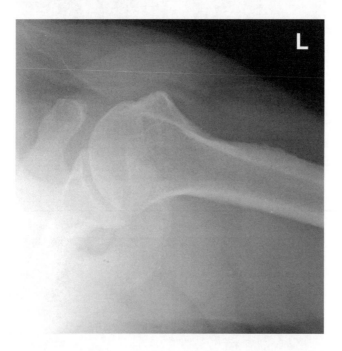

41. Figure 5-8: _____

_____

_____

Figure 5-9

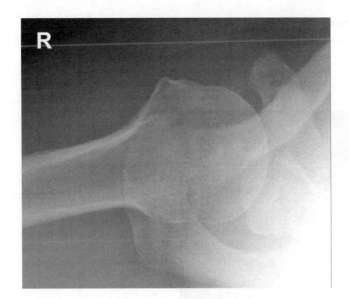

42. Figure 5-9: _____

_____

_____

Figure 5-10

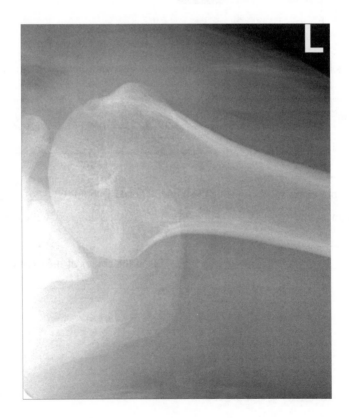

43. Figure 5-10: _____

_____

_____

44. Identify the labeled anatomy in Figure 5-11.

Figure 5-11

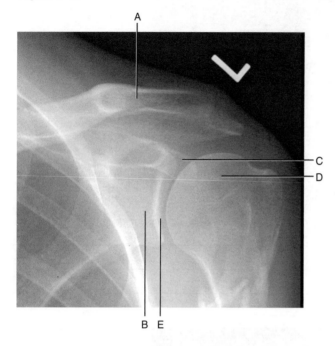

A. _____

B. _____

C. _____

D. _____

E. _____

45. Complete the statements below referring to AP oblique shoulder projection analysis guidelines.

AP Oblique (Grashey Method) Projection Analysis Guidelines
■ The glenoid cavity is demonstrated (A) _____, and the glenohumeral joint space is (B) _____.
■ The lateral coracoid process is superimposing the humeral head by about (C) _____.
■ The superior margin of the (D) _____ is aligned with the superior margin of the (E) _____.
■ The (F) _____ is at the center of the exposure field.

46. The (A) _____ and (B) _____ joints function coopera-
tively to allow the shoulder to be protracted.

47. The scapular body is positioned parallel with the IR for the AP oblique shoulder projection by aligning an imaginary

line connecting the (A) _____ and (B) _____ perpendicular to the IR.

48. A 45-degree oblique is routinely used for the AP oblique shoulder projection. List three situations in which the patient
requires more than 45 degrees of obliquity to obtain an AP oblique shoulder projection with accurate positioning.

A. _____

B. _____

C. _____

49. How is the clavicle positioned on an AP oblique shoulder projection with accurate rotation that was exposed with
the patient recumbent?

_____

50. Accurate CR centering on an AP oblique shoulder projection is accomplished by centering a (A) _____

CR to the (B) _____.

51. Which anatomic structures are demonstrated within the collimated field on an AP oblique shoulder projection with
accurate positioning?

_____

**For the following descriptions of AP oblique shoulder projections with poor positioning, state how the patient
would have been mispositioned for such a projection to be obtained.**

52. The glenohumeral joint space is closed, approximately 0.5 inch (1.25 cm) of the coracoid process is superimposed
over the humeral head, and the clavicle demonstrates excessive transverse foreshortening.

_____

53. The glenohumeral joint space is closed, the lateral tip of the coracoid process is not superimposed over the humeral
head, and the clavicle demonstrates little foreshortening.

_____

54. Recumbent patient: the glenohumeral joint is closed, and the clavicle is superimposed over the scapular neck.

_____

55. The superior margin of the coracoid process is demonstrated superior to the superior margin of the glenoid cavity.

_____

For the following AP oblique shoulder projections with poor positioning, state which anatomic structures are misaligned and how the patient should be repositioned for an optimal projection to be obtained.

Figure 5-12

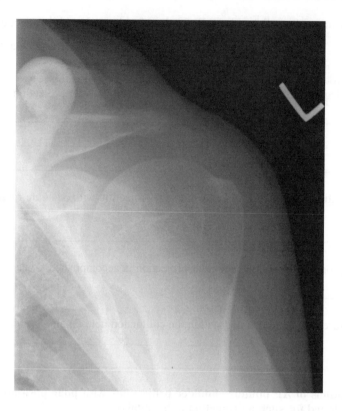

56. Figure 5-12: _____

_____

_____

Figure 5-13

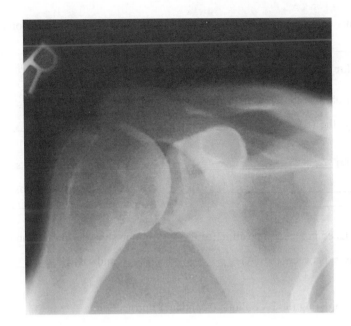

57. Figure 5-13: _____

_____

_____

Shoulder: PA Oblique Projection (Scapular Y)

58. Identify the labeled anatomy in Figure 5-14.

Figure 5-14

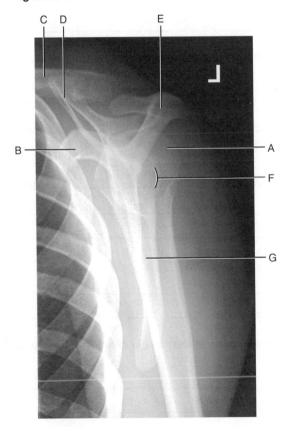

A. _____

B. _____

C. _____

D. _____

E. _____

F. _____

G. _____

59. Complete the statements below referring to PA oblique (scapular Y) shoulder projection analysis guidelines.

PA Oblique (Scapular Y) Shoulder Projection Analysis Guidelines
■ The lateral and vertebral scapular borders are (A) _____.
■ The scapular body, the (B) _____, and (C) _____ form a Y.
■ The clavicle and (D) _____ are visualized at the same transverse level.
■ The (E) _____ is at the center of the exposure field.

60. The scapular body is placed in a lateral position for the PA oblique shoulder projection by rotating the patient until an imaginary line drawn between the (A) _____ and (B) _____ is aligned parallel with the IR.

61. List two indications for ordering the PA oblique (scapular Y) projection:

    A. _____

    B. _____

62. For a PA oblique shoulder projection, the patient is rotated toward the (A) _____ (affected/unaffected) shoulder. For an AP oblique shoulder projection, the patient is rotated toward the (B) _____ (affected/unaffected) shoulder.

63. How can one distinguish the medial and lateral scapular borders from each other on a PA oblique shoulder projection with poor positioning?

    _____

64. Where are the humeral head and shaft positioned in respect to the scapula on a nondislocated PA oblique shoulder projection?

    _____

65. If the patient's shoulder is dislocated, should the Y formation desired on the PA oblique shoulder projection be visualized? _____ (Yes/No)

66. Where is the humeral head positioned on the AP oblique shoulder projection if the shoulder is dislocated anteriorly?

    A. _____

    _____

    If the shoulder is dislocated posteriorly?

    B. _____

    _____

67. How can the patient be positioned to prevent longitudinal foreshortening of the scapula on a PA oblique shoulder projection?

    _____

    _____

68. What spinal condition results in longitudinal scapular foreshortening on a PA oblique shoulder projection?

A. _____

How can the CR be adjusted to offset this foreshortening when obtaining a PA oblique projection?

B. _____

69. Accurate CR centering on a PA oblique shoulder projection is accomplished by centering a(n) (A) _____

CR to the (B) _____ border of the scapula halfway between the (C) _____ and

(D) _____.

70. Which anatomic structures are demonstrated on a PA oblique shoulder projection with accurate positioning?

_____

_____

For the following descriptions of PA oblique shoulder projections with poor positioning, state how the patient would have been mispositioned for such a projection to be obtained.

71. The vertebral and lateral borders of the scapular body are demonstrated without superimposition, the lateral scapular border is demonstrated next to the ribs, and the medial border appears laterally.

_____

_____

72. The lateral and medial borders of the scapula are demonstrated without superimposition, the thicker scapular border is demonstrated laterally, and the thinner scapular border is demonstrated next to the ribs.

_____

_____

73. The scapular body, acromion process, and coracoid process demonstrate a Y formation, but the superior scapular angle is demonstrated superior to the clavicle.

_____

_____

For the following AP oblique shoulder projections with poor positioning, state which anatomic structures are misaligned and how the patient should be repositioned for an optimal projection to be obtained.

Figure 5-15

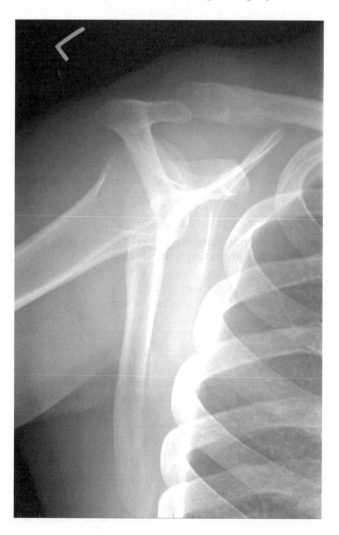

74. Figure 5-15: _____

_____

_____

Figure 5-16

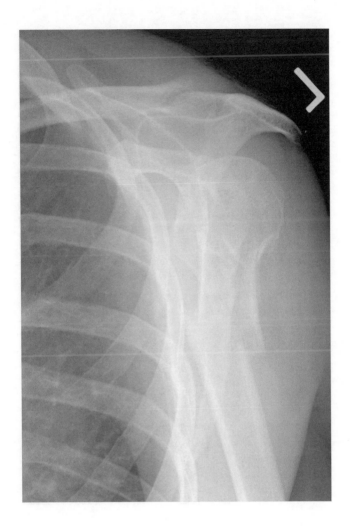

75. Figure 5-16, trauma: _____

_____

_____

Figure 5-17

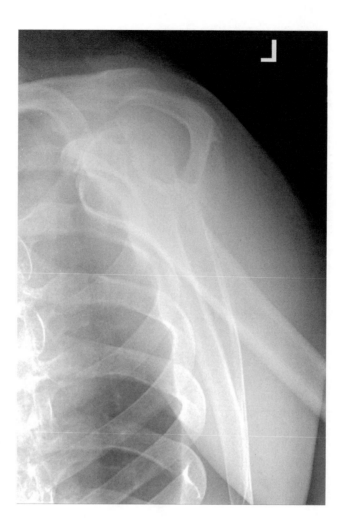

76. Figure 5-17: _____

_____

_____

Chapter **5** **Image Analysis of the Shoulder**

Figure 5-18

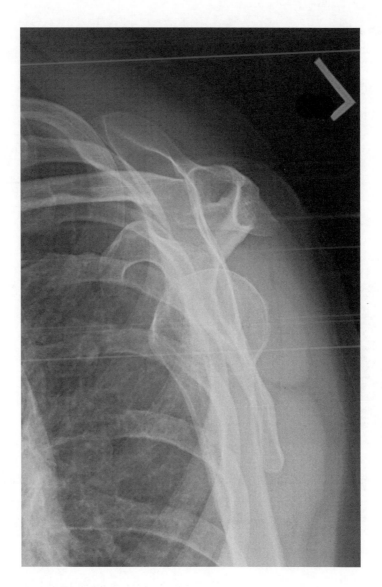

77. Figure 5-18: _____

_____

_____

Proximal Humerus: AP Axial Projection (Stryker "Notch" Method)

78. Identify the labeled anatomy in Figure 5-19.

Figure 5-19

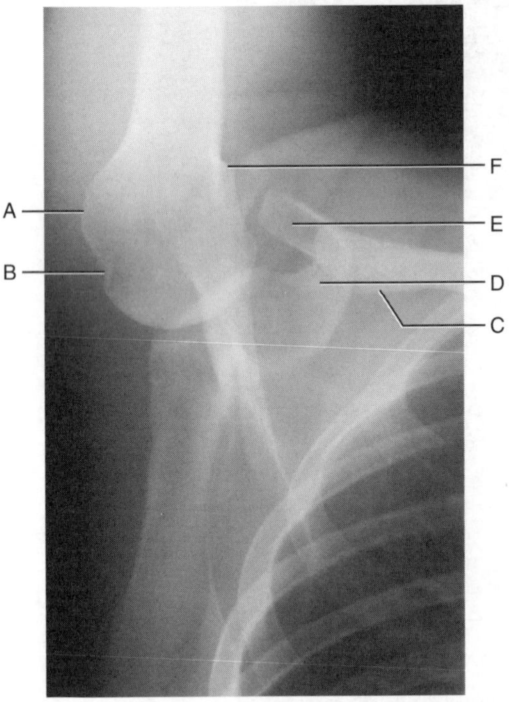

A. _____

B. _____

C. _____

D. _____

E. _____

F. _____

79. Complete the statements below referring to AP axial (Stryker notch) shoulder projection analysis guidelines.

AP Axial (Stryker "Notch" Method) Shoulder Projection Analysis Guidelines
■ The coracoid process is situated directly lateral to the (A) _____ of the clavicle.
■ The (B) _____ aspect of the humeral head is in profile laterally, and the greater and lesser tubercles are seen in partial profile.
■ The (C) _____ is superimposed over the lateral clavicle.
■ The (D) _____ is at the center of the exposure field.

80. The AP axial shoulder projection is performed to diagnose the presence of the (A) _____ defect of the shoulder. When present, the defect is demonstrated on the (B) _____ aspect of the humeral head.

81. For the AP axial shoulder projection, the affected arm is abducted until the humerus is (A) _____, and then the elbow is flexed and the palm of the hand is placed (B) _____.

82. Accurate CR centering on an AP axial projection is accomplished when the CR is centered to the _____
   _____.

83. Which anatomic structures are demonstrated on an AP axial projection with accurate positioning?

   _____

For the following descriptions of AP axial shoulder projections with poor positioning, state how the patient would have been mispositioned for such a projection to be obtained.

84. The coracoid process is seen inferior to the clavicle, and the humeral shaft demonstrates increased foreshortening.

_____

85. The lesser tubercle is seen in partial profile medially, but the greater tubercle and posterolateral humeral head are obscured.

_____

86. The posterolateral humeral head is obscured, and the humeral shaft demonstrates increased foreshortening.

_____

For the following AP axial shoulder projections with poor positioning, state which anatomic structures are misaligned and how the patient should be repositioned for an optimal projection to be obtained.

Figure 5-20

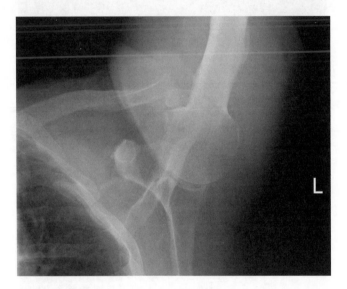

87. Figure 5-20: _____

_____

_____

Figure 5-21

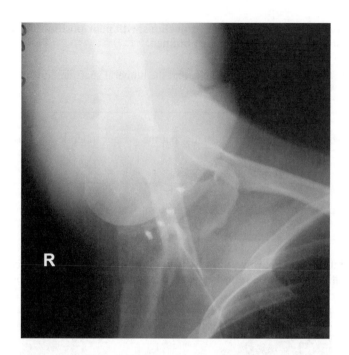

88. Figure 5-21: _____

_____

_____

Figure 5-22

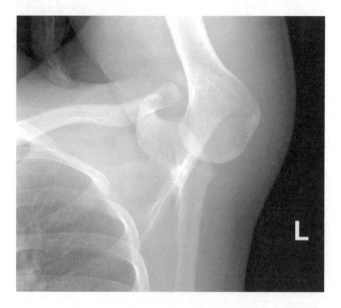

89. Figure 5-22: _____

_____

_____

Supraspinatus "Outlet": Tangential Projection (Neer Method)

90. Identify the labeled anatomy in Figure 5-23.

Figure 5-23

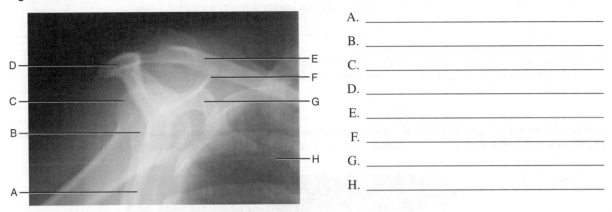

A. _____

B. _____

C. _____

D. _____

E. _____

F. _____

G. _____

H. _____

91. Complete the statements below referring to tangential supraspinatus outlet projection analysis guidelines.

Tangential "Outlet" Projection Analysis Guidelines

- The lateral and vertebral scapular borders are (A) _____.

- The (B) _____, (C) _____, and (D) _____ form a Y, with the glenoid cavity demonstrated on end.

- The lateral clavicle and acromion process form a smooth continuous arch, the superior scapular angle is at the level of the (E) _____ and is positioned about 0.5 inch (1.25 cm) inferior to the (F) _____.

- The (G) _____ is at the center of the exposure field.

---

92. Should the tangential outlet projection be obtained with the patient placed in an AP or PA oblique projection to demonstrate the least scapular magnification and the greatest scapular detail?

_____

93. Allowing the arm to dangle freely instead of keeping it abducted and flexed for the tangential outlet projection requires _____ (less/more) patient obliquity to obtain accurate positioning.

94. The tangential outlet projection is taken to identify spurs and osteophyte formation on the _____ surfaces of the lateral clavicle and acromion angle.

95. Accurate CR placement on a tangential outlet shoulder projection is accomplished when the CR is angled (A) _____ and centered to the (B) _____.

96. Which anatomic structures should be included within the collimated field?

_____

221

For the following descriptions of tangential outlet shoulder projections with poor positioning, state how the patient would have been mispositioned for such a projection to be obtained.

97. The vertebral and lateral borders of the scapular body are demonstrated without superimposition, the lateral scapular border is demonstrated next to the ribs, and the medial border appears laterally.

_____

98. The lateral clavicle and acromion process are demonstrated less than 0.5 inch (1.25 cm) superior to the humeral head and supraspinous fossa, and the superior scapular spine appears superior to the clavicle.

_____

For the following tangential outlet shoulder projections with poor positioning, state which anatomic structures are misaligned and how the patient should be repositioned for an optimal projection to be obtained.

Figure 5-24

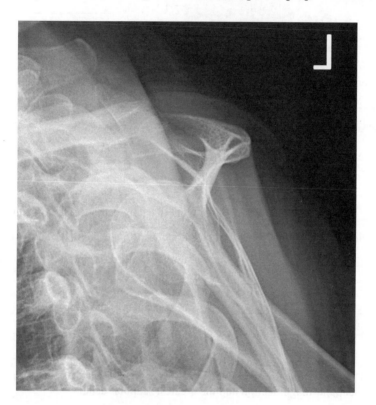

99. Figure 5-24: _____

_____

_____

Figure 5-25

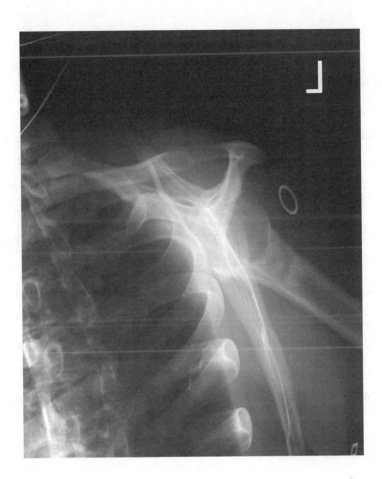

100. Figure 5-25: _____

_____

_____

Clavicle: AP Projection

101. Identify the labeled anatomy in Figure 5-26.

Figure 5-26

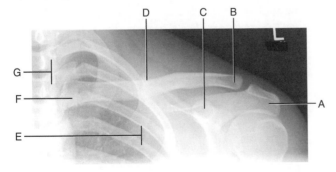

A. _____

B. _____

C. _____

D. _____

E. _____

F. _____

G. _____

102. Complete the statements below referring to AP clavicle projection analysis guidelines.

AP Clavicle Projection Analysis Guidelines

■ The medial clavicular end lies next to the (A) _____ of the vertebral column.

■ The clavicle and (B) _____ are visualized at the same

   (C) _____ level.

■ The (D) _____ is at the center of the exposure field.

---

103. How can the technologist position the patient to prevent rotation on an AP clavicular projection?

_____

104. Accurate CR centering on an AP clavicular is accomplished by centering a(n) (A) _____ CR to the

(B) _____.

105. Which anatomic structures are demonstrated on an AP clavicular projection with accurate positioning?

_____

For the following descriptions of AP clavicular projections with poor positioning, state how the patient would have been mispositioned for such a projection to be obtained.

106. The medial clavicular end is superimposed over the vertebral column, and the vertebral border of the scapula is positioned away from the thoracic cavity.

_____

107. The medial clavicular end is placed 1 inch (2.5 cm) away from the vertebral column, and the lateral border of the scapula is mostly superimposed by the thoracic cavity.

_____

108. The lateral clavicular end is superimposed over the scapular spine, and the superior scapular angle is projected above the midclavicle.

_____

For the following AP clavicular projections with poor positioning, state which anatomic structures are misaligned and how the patient should be repositioned for an optimal projection to be obtained.

Figure 5-27

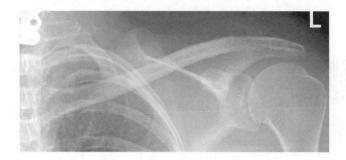

109. Figure 5-27: _____

_____

_____

Figure 5-28

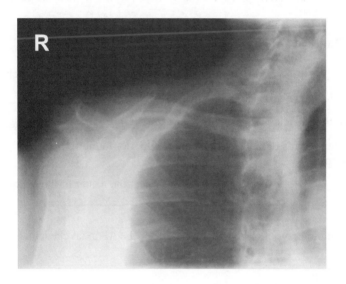

110. Figure 5-28: _____

_____

_____

Clavicle: AP Axial Projection (Lordotic Position)

111. Identify the labeled anatomy in Figure 5-29.

Figure 5-29

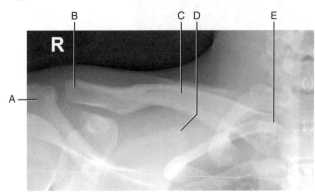

A. _____

B. _____

C. _____

D. _____

E. _____

112. Complete the statements below referring to AP axial clavicle projection analysis guidelines.

AP Axial Clavicle Projection Analysis Guidelines

■ The medial (A) _____ end lies next to the lateral edge of the vertebral column.

■ The superior scapular angle is visualized 0.5 inch (1.25 cm) (B) _____ to the clavicle.

■ The medial end of the clavicle is superimposed over the (C) _____ rib.

■ The middle and lateral thirds of the clavicle are seen superior to the (D) _____ and the clavicle bows upwardly.

■ The (E) _____ is at the center of the exposure field.

---

113. What are the degree and direction of CR angulation used for the AP axial clavicular projection?

_____

114. Where do most fractures of the clavicle occur?

_____

115. Which anatomic structures are demonstrated on an AP axial clavicular projection with accurate positioning?

_____

For the following descriptions of AP axial clavicular projections with poor positioning, state how the patient would have been mispositioned or the central ray aligned for such a projection to be obtained.

116. The medial clavicular end is drawn away from the vertebral column, the vertebral and lateral borders of the scapula are superimposed by the thoracic cavity, and the clavicle is longitudinally foreshortened.

_____

117. The lateral and middle thirds of the clavicle are superimposed over the scapula.

_____

For the following AP axial clavicular projection with poor positioning, state which anatomic structures are misaligned and how the patient should be repositioned for an optimal projection to be obtained.

Figure 5-30

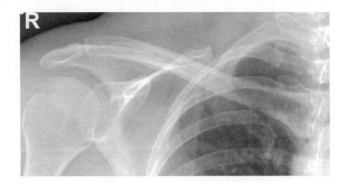

118. Figure 5-30: _____

_____

_____

AC Joint: AP Projection

119. Identify the labeled anatomy in Figure 5-31.

Figure 5-31

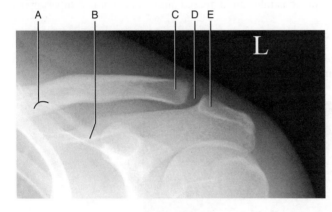

A. _____

B. _____

C. _____

D. _____

E. _____

120. Complete the statements below referring to AP acromioclavicular joint projection analysis guidelines.

AP Acromioclavicular Joint Projection Analysis Guidelines
■ Weight-bearing projection displays a (A) _____ marker to indicate that the projection was taken (B) _____. The lateral clavicle is (C) _____, and about 0.125 inch (0.3 cm) of space is present between the lateral clavicle and acromial apex.
■ The lateral clavicle demonstrates minimal (D) _____ superimposition.
■ The (E) _____ is at the center of the exposure field.

121. Why are weight- and non–weight-bearing AP AC joint projections often requested?

_____

_____

122. How is an AC ligament injury identified on an AP AC joint projection?

_____

_____

123. How much weight does the patient hold in each arm for the weight-bearing AC joint projection?

_____

124. Which anatomic structures are demonstrated on an AP AC joint projection with accurate positioning?

_____

125. Why is it necessary to place the CR at the same location when weight- and non–weight-bearing projections are requested?

_____

For the following description of an AP AC joint projection with poor positioning, state how the patient would have been mispositioned for such a projection to be obtained.

126. The left AC joint is closed, and the scapular body demonstrates an increased amount of thoracic superimposition.

_____

For the following AC joint projection with poor positioning, state which anatomic structures are misaligned and how the patient should be repositioned for an optimal projection to be obtained.

Figure 5-32

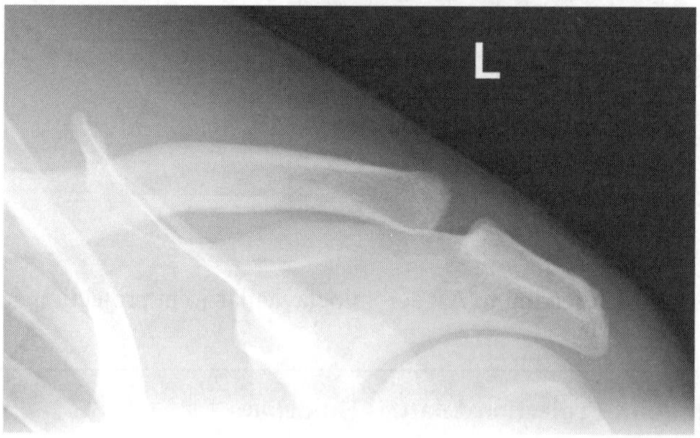

127. Figure 5-32: _____

_____

_____

Scapula: AP Projection

128. Identify the labeled anatomy in Figure 5-33.

Figure 5-33

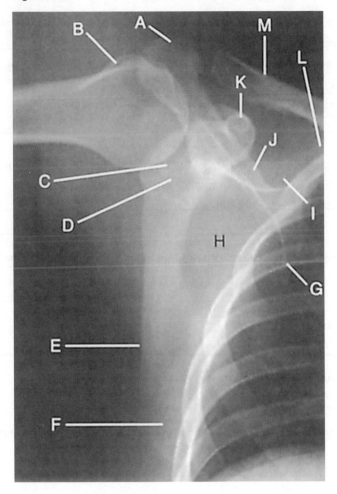

A. _____

B. _____

C. _____

D. _____

E. _____

F. _____

G. _____

H. _____

I. _____

J. _____

K. _____

L. _____

M. _____

129. Complete the statements below referring to AP scapula projection analysis guidelines.

AP Scapula Projection Analysis Guidelines
■ The anterior and posterior margins of the (A) _____ are nearly superimposed.
■ The superior scapular angle is about 0.25 inch (0.6 cm) inferior to the (B) _____.
■ The lateral border of the scapula is seen without (C) _____ superimposition, and the thoracic cavity is superimposing the (D) _____.
■ The (E) _____ is at the center of the exposure field.

130. Even though the AP thickness is approximately the same across the scapula, why is the brightness level not uniform across the scapula?

_____

_____

131. What degree of scapular rotation is demonstrated when the patient is positioned in an AP projection with the humerus resting against the side?

A. _____

Which scapular dimension is foreshortened in this position?

B. _____

132. How is the patient's arm positioned for an AP projection of the scapula?

A. _____

What effect does this positioning have on the shoulder when the projection is obtained with the patient in a supine position?

B. _____

What effect does the positioning have on the visualization of the glenoid cavity on an AP scapular projection?

C. _____

133. What scapular dimension is foreshortened when the patient's midcoronal plane is poorly positioned?

_____

134. Accurate CR centering on an AP scapular projection is accomplished by centering a (A) _____ CR (B) _____ inch(es) (C) _____ to the palpable coracoid process.

135. Which anatomic structures are included on an AP scapular projection with accurate positioning?

_____

For the following descriptions of AP scapular projections with poor positioning, state how the patient would have been mispositioned for such a projection to be obtained.

136. The glenoid cavity is not in profile, and approximately 0.5 inch (1.25 cm) of it is demonstrated.

_____

137. A projection of a patient who was very mobile demonstrates the inferior scapular angle and inferolateral scapular border with thoracic cavity superimposition.

_____

For the following AP scapular projections with poor positioning, state which anatomic structures are misaligned and how the patient should be repositioned for an optimal projection to be obtained.

Figure 5-34

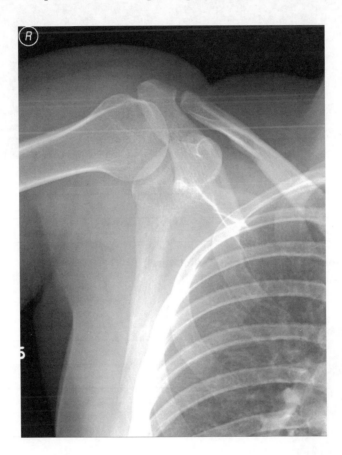

138. Figure 5-34: _____

_____

_____

Figure 5-35

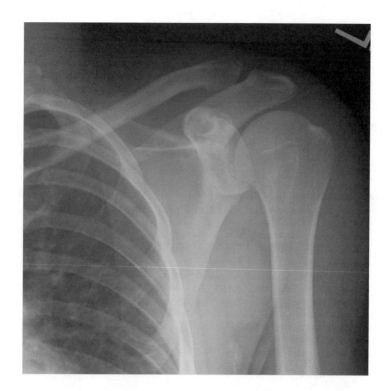

139. Figure 5-35: _____

_____

_____

Scapula: Lateral Projection (Lateromedial or Mediolateral)

140. Identify the labeled anatomy in Figure 5-36.

Figure 5-36

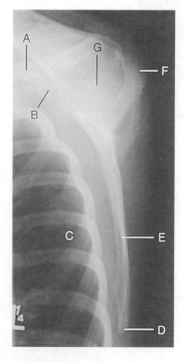

A. _____

B. _____

C. _____

D. _____

E. _____

F. _____

G. _____

141. Complete the statements below referring to lateral scapula projection analysis guidelines.

Lateral Scapula Projection Analysis Guidelines
■ The superior scapular angle is just inferior to the (A) _____ .
■ The lateral and vertebral scapular borders are (B) _____.
■ The (C) _____ is at the center of the exposure field.

142. The lateral scapula is positioned with the patient placed in an AP or PA oblique projection. For the AP oblique projection, the patient is rotated (A) _____ (toward/away from) the affected scapula, and for the PA oblique projection, the patient is rotated (B) _____ (toward/away from) the affected scapula.

143. What patient positioning procedure determines the degree of obliquity needed to place the scapula in a lateral position?

_____

144. How is rotation identified on a lateral scapular projection with poor positioning?

_____

145. Most scapular fractures occur at the (A) _____ and (B) _____ of the scapula.

146. What humeral position with respect to the body places the long axis of the scapula parallel with the IR for a lateral scapular projection?

_____

_____

147. What humeral position with respect to the body places the lateral border of the scapula parallel with the IR for a lateral scapular projection?

_____

_____

148. The higher the humerus is elevated for a lateral scapular projection, the (A) _____ (more/less) the patient needs to be rotated to obtain accurate positioning. Why? (B) _____

149. Which anatomic structures are included on a lateral scapular projection with accurate positioning?

_____

_____

For the following descriptions of lateral scapular projections with poor positioning, state how the patient would have been mispositioned for such a projection to be obtained.

150. The lateral and vertebral borders of the scapula are demonstrated without superimposition, the thick border is next to the ribs, and the thin border is demonstrated laterally.

_____

151. The lateral and vertebral borders of the scapula are demonstrated without superimposition, the lateral border is demonstrated laterally, and the vertebral border appears next to the ribs.

_____

_____

For the following lateral scapular projections with poor positioning, state which anatomic structures are misaligned and how the patient should be repositioned for an optimal projection to be obtained.

Figure 5-37

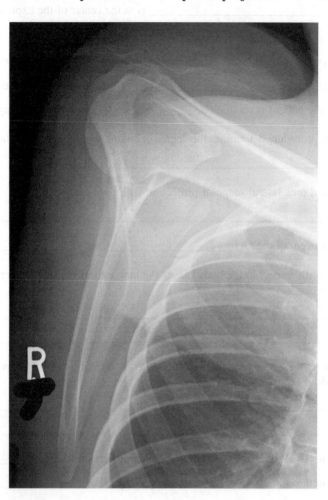

152. Figure 5-37: _____

_____

_____

Figure 5-38

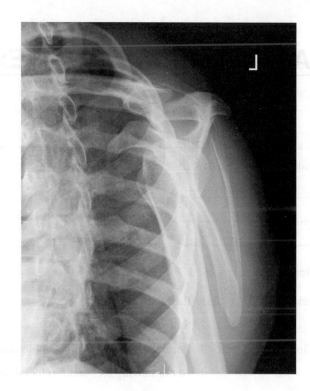

153. Figure 5-38: _____

_____

_____

6 Image Analysis of the Lower Extremity

STUDY QUESTIONS

1. State the kV range for the following projections.

   A. Lateral ankle: _____

   B. Grid, AP knee: _____

   C. AP femur: _____

2. Match the term with its definition.

   _____ A. Abductor tubercle   1. Partial dislocation

   _____ B. Dorsiflex   2. Sole of foot

   _____ C. Intermalleolar line   3. Located posteriorly on medial femoral condyle

   _____ D. Lateral mortise   4. Act of moving toes and forefoot downward

   _____ E. Plantar   5. Lateral side of knee joint is narrower

   _____ F. Plantar flexion   6. Opening between the calcaneus and talus

   _____ G. Subluxation   7. Line connecting medial and lateral malleoli

   _____ H. Tarsi sinus   8. Medial side of knee joint narrower

   _____ I. Valgus deformity   9. Act of moving toes and forefoot upward

   _____ J. Varus deformity   10. Tibiofibular joint

Toe: AP Axial Projection

3. Identify the labeled anatomy in Figure 6-1.

Figure 6-1

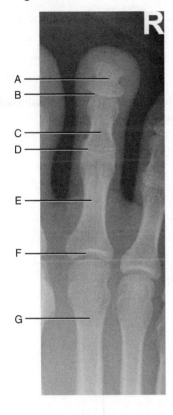

A. _____

B. _____

C. _____

D. _____

E. _____

F. _____

G. _____

4. Complete the statements below referring to AP axial toe projection analysis guidelines.

AP Axial Toe(s) Projection Analysis Guidelines

- The (A) _____ width and midshaft (B) _____ are equal on both sides of phalanges.

- The (C) _____ and (D) _____ joints are open, and the phalanges are seen without foreshortening.

- The (E) _____ joint is at the center of the exposure field for a toe projection and

  (F) _____ MTP joint is at the center when all toes are imaged.

---

5. If the toe is medially rotated for a right AP axial toe projection, the (A) _____ (medial/lateral)

   side of the toe demonstrates the greatest soft tissue width, and the (B) _____ (medial/lateral) side demonstrates the greatest phalangeal midshaft concavity.

6. To obtain open joint spaces on an AP axial toe projection, align the CR (A) _____ to the joint space and align the joint space (B) _____ to the IR.

7. Which anatomic structures are included on an AP axial toe projection with accurate positioning?

_____

237

For the following descriptions of AP axial toe projections with poor positioning, state how the patient would have been mispositioned for such a projection to be obtained.

8. The phalanges demonstrate more soft tissue width on the medial toe surface than on the lateral surface.

_____

9. The IP and MTP joint spaces are closed, and the phalanges are foreshortened.

_____

For the following AP axial toe projections with poor positioning, state which anatomic structures are misaligned and how the patient should be repositioned for an optimal projection to be obtained.

Figure 6-2

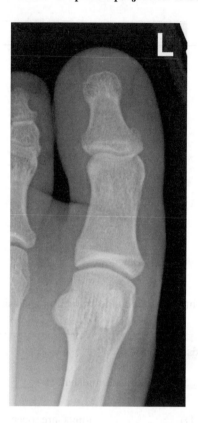

10. Figure 6-2: _____

_____

_____

_____

Toe: AP Oblique Projection

11. Identify the labeled anatomy in Figure 6-3.

Figure 6-3

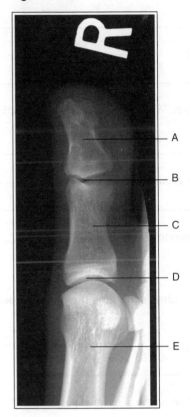

A. _____

B. _____

C. _____

D. _____

E. _____

12. Complete the statements below referring to AP oblique toe projection analysis guidelines.

AP Oblique Toe(s) Projection Analysis Guidelines
■ (A) _____ as much soft tissue width and more phalangeal concavity are present on the side of the digit rotated (B)(away from/toward) _____ the IR.
■ The (C) _____ and (D) _____ joint(s) are open, and the phalanges are demonstrated without foreshortening.
■ (E) _____ joint is at the center of the exposure field for a toe projection, and the third MTP joint is at the center when all toes are imaged.

13. What degree of patient toe obliquity is used for an AP oblique toe projection?

A. _____

How is the accuracy of the degree of toe obliquity identified on an AP oblique toe projection?

B. _____

14. In what direction are the foot and toe rotated for a first through third AP oblique toe projection?

A. _____

For a fourth through fifth AP oblique toe projection?

B. _____

Why are the patient's foot and toe rotated differently for these examinations?

C. _____

15. The patient was unable to fully extend the toe for an AP oblique toe projection. What will the resulting projection demonstrate if a perpendicular CR was used for this patient?

_____

16. Which anatomic structures are included on an AP oblique toe projection with accurate positioning?

_____

17. Why is it important to not have soft tissue overlap on an AP oblique toe projection?_____

_____.

For the following descriptions of AP oblique toe projections with poor positioning, state how the patient would have been mispositioned for such a projection to be obtained.

18. The soft tissue width demonstrated on each side of the phalanges is nearly equal.

_____

19. The proximal phalanx demonstrates more concavity on the posterior aspect than on the anterior aspect.

_____

20. The IP and MTP joint spaces are obscured and the phalanges foreshortened.

_____

For the following AP oblique toe projections with poor positioning, state which anatomic structures are misaligned and how the patient should be repositioned for such a projection to be obtained.

Figure 6-4

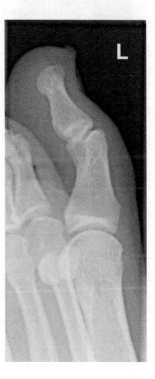

21. Figure 6-4: _____

_____

_____

_____

Figure 6-5

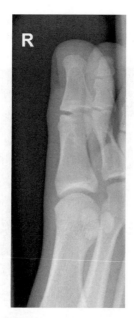

22. Figure 6-5: _____

_____

_____

_____

Figure 6-6

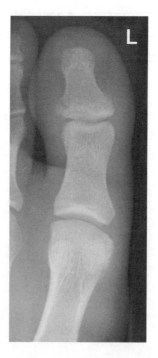

23. Figure 6-6: _____

_____

_____

_____

Toe: Lateral Projection

24. Identify the labeled anatomy in Figure 6-7.

Figure 6-7

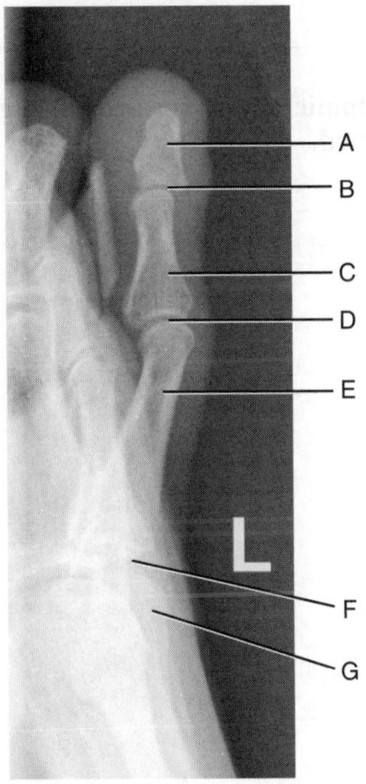

A. _____

B. _____

C. _____

D. _____

E. _____

F. _____

G. _____

25. Complete the statements below referring to lateral toe projection analysis guidelines.

Lateral Toe Projection Analysis Guidelines
■ The (A) _____ of the proximal phalanx are superimposed.
■ There is no (B) _____ or bony overlap from adjacent toes.
■ The (C) _____ joint is at the center of the exposure field.

26. To position the toe in a lateral projection, the foot is rotated (A) _____ (medially/laterally) when the first, second, and third toes are imaged and (B) _____ (medially/laterally) when the fourth and fifth toes are imaged.

27. Which anatomic structures are included on a lateral toe projection with accurate positioning?

_____

For the following descriptions of lateral toe projections with poor positioning, state how the patient would have been mispositioned for such a projection to be obtained.

28. The proximal phalanx demonstrates nearly equal midshaft concavity, and the MT heads are demonstrated posterior to the first toe.

_____

243

29. The condyles of the proximal phalanx are shown without superimposition, and the MT heads are superimposed.

_____

30. Soft tissue and bony overlap of unaffected digits onto the affected digit is present.

_____

For the following lateral toe projections with poor positioning, state which anatomic structures are misaligned and how the patient should be repositioned for an optimal projection to be obtained.

Figure 6-8

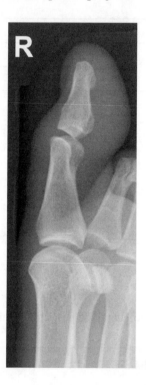

31. Figure 6-8: _____

_____

_____

_____

Figure 6-9

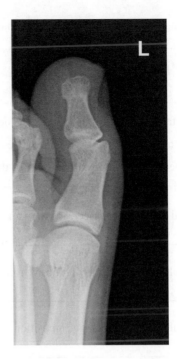

32. Figure 6-9: _____

_____

_____

_____

Foot: AP Axial Projection (Dorsoplantar Projection)

33. Identify the labeled anatomy in Figure 6-10.

Figure 6-10

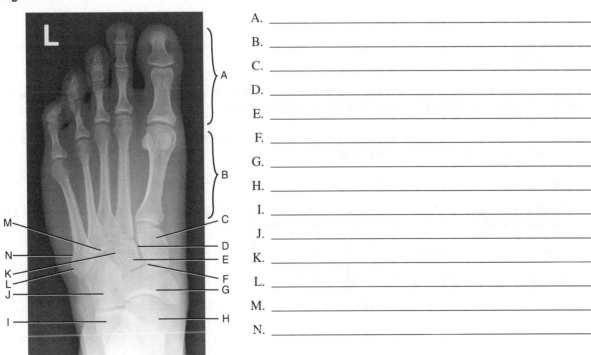

A. _____

B. _____

C. _____

D. _____

E. _____

F. _____

G. _____

H. _____

I. _____

J. _____

K. _____

L. _____

M. _____

N. _____

34. Complete the statements below referring to AP axial foot projection analysis guidelines.

AP Axial Foot Projection Analysis Guidelines

- Joint space between the (A) _____ and (B) _____ cuneiforms is open, and about

  (C) _____ of the talus is superimposing the calcaneus.
- (D) _____ and navicular–cuneiform joint spaces are open.
- (E) _____ metatarsal base is at the center of the exposure field.

35. For an AP axial foot projection, equal pressure is placed on the (A) _____ foot surface, and the

    (B) _____, (C) _____, and (D) _____ should remain aligned.

36. Will medial or lateral foot rotation result in the talus moving away from the calcaneus?

    _____

37. Will medial or lateral foot rotation result in increased superimposition of the MT bases?

    _____

38. A(n) (A) _____ degree proximal CR angulation is required for an AP axial foot projection to demonstrate open TMT joint spaces. Is a higher degree of CR angulation needed in a patient with a low medial

    longitudinal arch or a high medial longitudinal arch? (B) _____

39. Which anatomic structures are included on an AP axial foot projection with accurate positioning?

    _____

40. Why are weight-bearing projections of the foot obtained?

    _____

41. On a weight-bearing AP foot, the CR angulation needed may be less than what is needed for a non–weight-bearing AP foot. Why? _____

For the following descriptions of AP axial foot projections with poor positioning, state how the patient or CR would have been mispositioned for such a projection to be obtained.

42. The joint space between the medial and intermediate cuneiforms is closed, the navicular is demonstrated in profile, and more than one-third of the talus superimposes the calcaneus.

    _____

43. The joint space between the medial and intermediate cuneiforms is closed, the calcaneus is demonstrated without talar superimposition, and the MT bases demonstrate decreased superimposition.

    _____

44. The TMT and navicular–cuneiform joint spaces are obscured.

    _____

For the following AP axial foot projections with poor positioning, state which anatomic structures are misaligned and how the patient should be repositioned for an optimal projection to be obtained.

Figure 6-11

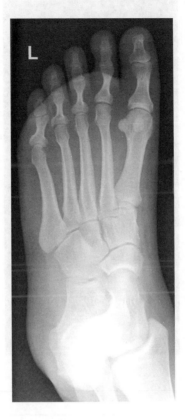

45. Figure 6-11: _____

_____

_____

_____

Figure 6-12

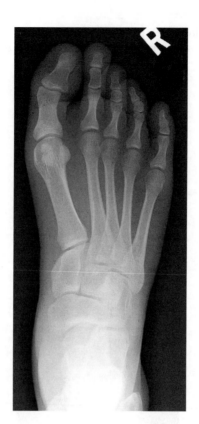

46. Figure 6-12: _____
_____
_____
_____

Foot: AP Oblique Projection (Medial Rotation)

47. Identify the labeled anatomy in Figure 6-13.

Figure 6-13

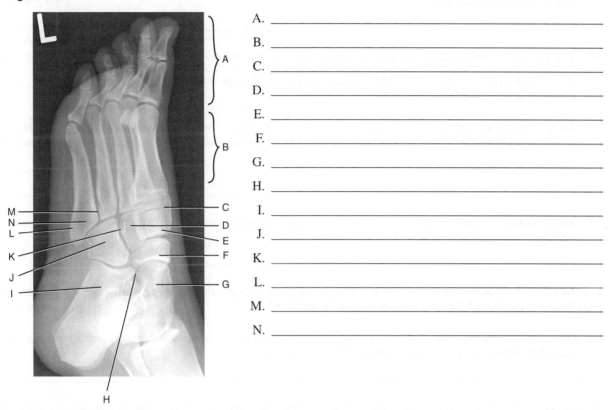

A. _____

B. _____

C. _____

D. _____

E. _____

F. _____

G. _____

H. _____

I. _____

J. _____

K. _____

L. _____

M. _____

N. _____

48. Complete the statements below referring to AP oblique foot projection analysis guidelines.

AP Oblique Foot Projection Analysis Guidelines

- The (A) _____ and the (B) _____ intermetatarsal joints spaces are open.

- Tarsi sinus and (C) _____ metatarsal tuberosity are visualized.

- (D) _____ base is at the center of the exposure field.

---

49. An AP oblique foot projection is obtained by rotating the patient 30 to 60 degrees _____ (medially/laterally).

50. The degree of foot obliquity needed for an AP oblique foot projection varies according to the height of the medial longitudinal arch. What degree of obliquity is used in a patient with a high medial longitudinal arch?

A. _____

In a patient with a low medial longitudinal arch?

B. _____

In a patient with an average medial longitudinal arch?

C. _____

249

51. View the AP oblique foot projection in Figure 6-13. State whether the patient has a high or low medial longitudinal arch.

A. _____

How did you determine this?

B. _____

52. As a foot is rotated medially from an AP projection, the first MT base rotates (A) _____ (over/ beneath) the (B) _____ MT base and the second through third MT heads move (C) _____ (closer to/farther away from) one another.

53. When the foot is medially rotated more than needed for an AP oblique foot projection with accurate positioning, will the fourth MT tubercle be superimposed over the fifth MT or will the fifth MT be superimposed over the fourth MT?

_____

_____

54. Which anatomic structures are demonstrated within the collimated field on an AP oblique foot projection with accurate positioning?

_____

For the following descriptions of AP oblique foot projections with poor positioning, state how the patient would have been mispositioned for such a projection to be obtained.

55. The lateral cuneiform–cuboid, navicular–cuboid, and third through fifth intermetatarsal spaces are closed, and the fourth MT tubercle is demonstrated without fifth MT superimposition.

_____

56. The lateral cuneiform–cuboid, navicular–cuboid, and intermetatarsal joint spaces are closed, and the fifth MT is superimposed over the fourth MT tubercle.

_____

For the following AP oblique foot projection with poor positioning, state which anatomic structures are misaligned and how the patient should be repositioned for an optimal projection to be obtained.

Figure 6-14

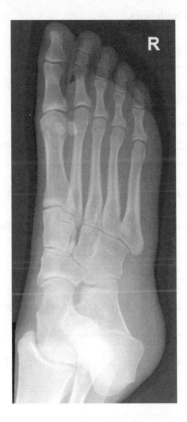

57. Figure 6-14: _____

_____

_____

_____

Foot: Lateral Projection (Mediolateral and Lateromedial)

58. Identify the labeled anatomy in Figure 6-15.

Figure 6-15

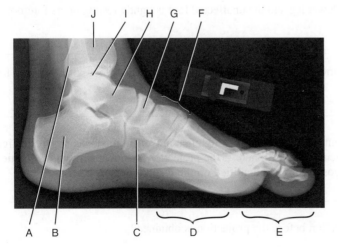

A. _____

B. _____

C. _____

D. _____

E. _____

F. _____

G. _____

H. _____

I. _____

J. _____

59. Complete the statements below referring to lateral foot projection analysis guidelines.

Lateral Foot Projection Analysis Guidelines
■ Contrast and density are adequate to demonstrate the (A) _____ and (B) _____ fat pads.
■ Proximal talar domes are aligned, the (C) _____ joint is open, and the distal fibula is super-imposed by the posterior half of the distal tibia.
■ The long axis of the foot is positioned at a (D) _____ angle with the lower leg.
■ (E) _____ are at the center of the exposure field.

60. Which surface of the foot is positioned against the IR for a mediolateral projection of the foot? _____

61. List the two soft tissue fat pads that should be demonstrated on a lateral foot projection, and describe their locations.

A. _____

B. _____

62. How is the lower leg placed to obtain a lateral foot projection with accurate positioning?

_____

63. How is the foot positioned with the lower leg and IR to obtain a lateral foot projection with accurate positioning?

A. Lower leg: _____

B. IR: _____

64. How do the following foot and lower leg positions affect the COG (center of gravity) and BOS (base of support)?

A. Affected foot at an 85-degree angle with the lower leg when the unaffected foot is in front of the affected foot and 95-degree angle with the lower leg when the unaffected foot is in back of the affected foot:

_____

B. Affected foot at a 100-degree angle with the lower leg and was obtained with the unaffected foot positioned too far behind the affected foot:

_____

C. Affected foot is at a 90-degree angle with the lower leg and the unaffected foot is lightly resting on its forefoot or toes:

_____

D. Affected foot is at a 75-degree angle with the lower leg and was taken with the unaffected foot positioned too far in front of the affected foot:

_____

65. A lateral foot projection was requested for a patient with a large upper thigh that prevented the lower leg from align-ing parallel with the imaging table when the patient was positioned. If the projection was obtained with the patient positioned in this manner, how would this poor positioning be identified on the resulting projection?

A. _____

How is the positioning setup adjusted in this situation before the projection is obtained?

B. _____

252

66. The height of the medial longitudinal arch can be determined on a lateral foot projection with accurate positioning by measuring the amount of cuboid that appears (A) _____ to the (B) _____.

67. The average lateral foot projection demonstrates approximately _____ inch(es) of the cuboid posterior to the navicular.

68. In a patient with a low medial foot arch, (A) _____ (more/less) of the cuboid will be demonstrated posterior to the navicular, and in a patient with a high medial foot arch, (B) _____ (more/less) will be demonstrated.

69. View the lateral foot projections in Figures 6-15 and 6-17. State which projection was obtained from the patient with the higher medial longitudinal arch.

    A. _____

    How did you determine this difference?

    B. _____

70. Misalignment of the talar domes can be caused by poor (A) _____ or (B) _____ positioning.

71. If the distal tibia is positioned farther from the imaging table than the proximal tibia for a lateral foot projection, the (A) _____ (lateral/medial) dome is demonstrated (B) _____ to the (C) _____ (lateral/medial) talar dome and the medial foot arch appears (D) _____ (higher/lower) on the resulting projection.

72. If the proximal tibia is positioned farther from the imaging table than the distal tibia for a lateral foot projection, the (A) _____ dome is demonstrated (B) _____ to the (C) _____ talar dome, and the medial foot arch appears (D) _____ (higher/lower) on the resulting projection.

73. If a lateral foot projection with poor positioning demonstrates an obscured tibiotalar joint space, one talar dome proximal to the other, and the navicular superimposed over most of the cuboid, which dome is proximal?

    _____

74. If the calcaneus is positioned too close to the IR and the forefoot is raised off the IR for a lateral foot projection, the (A) _____ talar dome is demonstrated (B) _____ to the (C) _____ talar dome, and the fibula is demonstrated too far (D) _____ on the tibia.

75. If the forefoot is positioned too close to the IR and the calcaneus is elevated off the IR for a lateral foot projection, the (A) _____ talar dome is demonstrated (B) _____ to the (C) _____ talar dome, and the fibula is demonstrated too far (D) _____ on the tibia.

76. Why is it important to dorsiflex the foot to a 90-degree angle with the lower leg?

    A. _____

    B. _____

    C. _____

77. Against which aspect of the foot is the IR placed for a standing lateromedial projection of the foot?

A. _____

Which surface (medial/lateral) of the foot is aligned parallel with the IR for a lateromedial projection of the foot with accurate positioning?

B. _____

78. If a standing lateromedial projection of the foot with poor positioning demonstrates one talar dome posterior to the other talar dome and the fibula is situated too far posterior on the tibia, how should the patient's position be adjusted for an optimal projection to be obtained?

_____

79. Accurate CR centering on a lateral foot projection is accomplished by centering a(n) (A) _____ CR

to the foot midline at the level of the (B) _____ .

80. Which anatomic structures are included on a lateral foot projection with accurate positioning?

_____

For the following descriptions of mediolateral foot projections with poor positioning, state how the patient would have been mispositioned for such a projection to be obtained.

81. The tibiotalar joint space is obscured, one talar dome is demonstrated proximal to the other dome, and the navicular is superimposed over most of the cuboid.

_____

82. The tibiotalar joint space is obscured, one talar dome is demonstrated proximal to the other dome, and more than 0.5 inch (1.25 cm) of the cuboid appears posterior to the navicular.

_____

83. The tibiotalar joint is obscured, one talar dome is demonstrated anterior to the other dome, and the fibula is demonstrated too posterior on the tibia.

_____

84. The tibiotalar joint is obscured, one talar dome is demonstrated anterior to the other dome, and the fibula is demonstrated too anterior on the tibia.

_____

For the following lateral foot projections with poor positioning, state which anatomic structures are misaligned and how the patient should be repositioned for an optimal projection to be obtained.

Figure 6-16

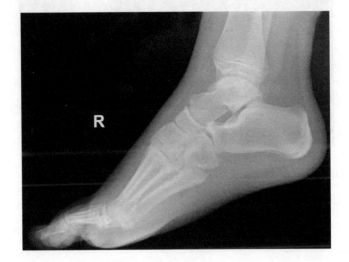

85. Figure 6-16: _____

_____

_____

_____

Figure 6-17

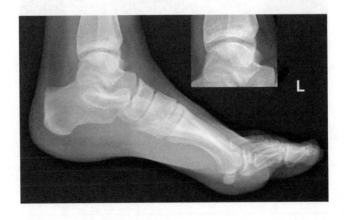

86. Figure 6-17: _____

_____

_____

_____

Chapter **6** **Image Analysis of the Lower Extremity**

Figure 6-18

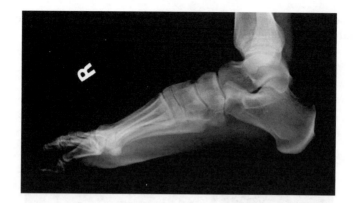

87. Figure 6-18, mediolateral projection, average medial arch:

_____

_____

_____

Figure 6-19

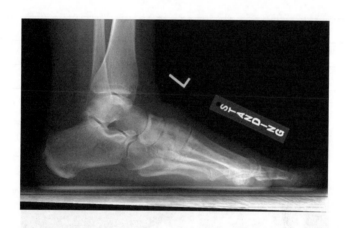

88. Figure 6-19, lateromedial projection:

_____

_____

_____

Calcaneus: Axial Projection (Plantodorsal)

89. Identify the labeled anatomy in Figure 6-20.

Figure 6-20

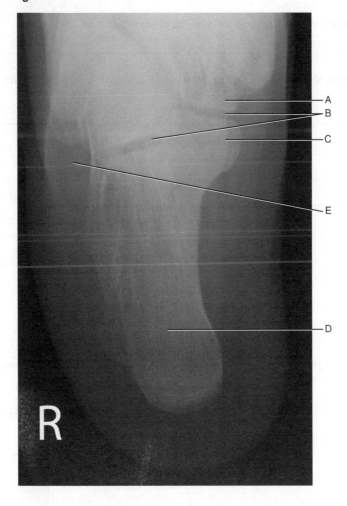

A. _____

B. _____

C. _____

D. _____

E. _____

90. Complete the statements below referring to axial calcaneus projection analysis guidelines.

Axial Calcaneus Projection Analysis Guidelines
■ The (A) _____ joint is open, and the calcaneal tuberosity is demonstrated with minimal distortion.
■ The second through fourth distal MTs are not demonstrated on the (B) _____ or (C) _____ aspects of the foot, respectively.
■ The (D) _____ is at the center of the exposure field.

91. To obtain an axial calcaneal projection with accurate positioning, position the foot (A) _____ and direct a (B) _____-degree proximal CR angulation toward the (C) _____ foot surface.

92. When the CR and foot are accurately aligned, the CR is aligned (A) _____ to the talocalcaneal joint space and (B) _____ to the calcaneal tuberosity.

257

93. If an axial calcaneal projection is requested for a patient who is unable to dorsiflex the foot to a vertical position, how is the positioning setup adjusted before the projection is obtained?

A. _____

How is the setup changed if the patient dorsiflexed the foot beyond the vertical position?

B. _____

94. Which anatomic structures can be used to estimate the CR angulation needed when the patient is unable to dorsiflex the foot into a vertical position?

_____

95. How is the patient positioned to prevent calcaneal tilting?

A. _____

How is calcaneal tilting identified on an axial calcaneal projection with poor positioning?

B. _____

96. Accurate CR centering on an axial calcaneal projection is accomplished by centering the CR to the midline of the foot at the level of the _____.

97. Which anatomic structures are included on an axial calcaneal projection with accurate positioning?

_____

For the following descriptions of axial calcaneal projections with poor positioning, state how the patient would have been mispositioned for such a projection to be obtained.

98. The talocalcaneal joint space is obscured, and the calcaneal tuberosity is foreshortened. The standard 40-degree angulation was used.

_____

99. The first MT is demonstrated medially.

_____

100. The fourth and fifth MTs are demonstrated laterally.

_____

For the following axial calcaneal projection with poor positioning, state which anatomic structures are misaligned and how the patient should be repositioned for an optimal projection to be obtained.

Figure 6-21

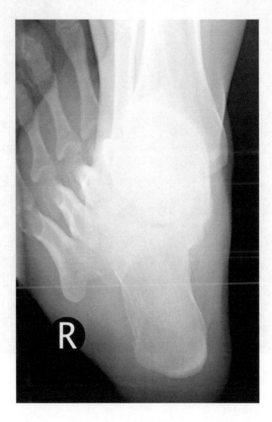

101. Figure 6-21: _____

_____

_____

_____

Figure 6-22

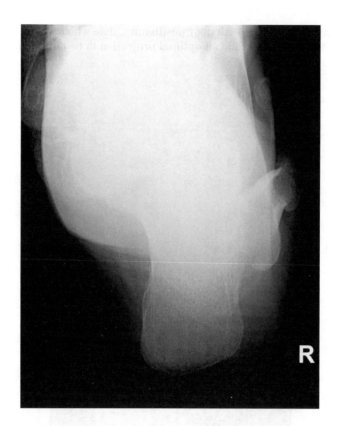

102. Figure 6-22: _____

_____

_____

_____

Figure 6-23

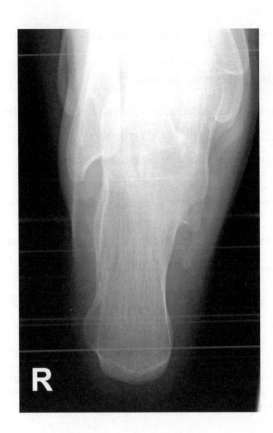

103. Figure 6-23: _____

_____

_____

_____

Calcaneus: Lateral Projection (Mediolateral)

104. Identify the labeled anatomy in Figure 6-24.

Figure 6-24

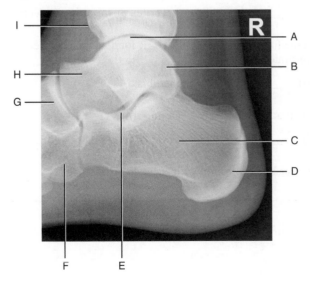

A. _____

B. _____

C. _____

D. _____

E. _____

F. _____

G. _____

H. _____

I. _____

105. Complete the statements below referring to lateral calcaneus projection analysis guidelines.

> **Lateral Calcaneus Projection Analysis Guidelines**
>
> - The talar domes are superimposed, the tibiotalar joint space is open, and the distal fibula is superimposed by the (A) _____ half of the distal tibia.
> - The long axis of the foot is positioned at a 90-degree angle with the (B) _____.
> - The (C) _____ is at the center of the exposure field.

106. How is the lower leg positioned to obtain a lateral calcaneal projection with accurate positioning?

_____

107. How is the foot positioned with the lower leg and IR to obtain a lateral calcaneal projection with accurate positioning?

A. Lower leg: _____

B. IR: _____

108. A calcaneal foot projection was requested for a patient with a large upper thigh that prevented the lower leg from aligning parallel with the imaging table when the patient was positioned. If the projection was obtained with the patient positioned in this manner, how would this poor positioning be identified on the resulting projection?

_____

109. The height of the medial longitudinal arch is determined on a lateral calcaneal projection with accurate positioning by measuring the amount of cuboid that appears (A) _____ to the (B) _____.

110. The average calcaneal projection demonstrates approximately _____ inch(es) of the cuboid posterior to the navicular.

111. If the distal tibia is positioned farther from the imaging table than the proximal tibia for a lateral calcaneal projection, the (A) _____ dome is demonstrated (B) _____ to the (C) _____ talar dome, and the medial longitudinal foot arch appears (D) _____ (higher/lower) on the resulting projection.

112. If the calcaneus is positioned too close to the IR and the forefoot is raised off the IR for a lateral calcaneal projection, the (A) _____ talar dome is demonstrated (B) _____ to the (C) _____ talar dome, and the fibula is demonstrated too far (D) _____ on the tibia.

113. Accurate CR centering on a lateral calcaneal projection is accomplished by centering a(n) (A) _____ CR 1 inch (2.5 cm) (B) _____ to the (C) _____.

114. Which anatomic structures are included on a lateral calcaneal projection with accurate positioning?

_____

For the following descriptions of lateral calcaneal projections with poor positioning, state how the patient would have been mispositioned for such a projection to be obtained.

115. The tibiotalar joint space is obscured, one talar dome is demonstrated proximal to the other, and the navicular bone is superimposed over most of the cuboid.

_____

116. The tibiotalar joint is obscured, one talar dome is demonstrated anterior to the other dome, and the fibula is demonstrated too posterior on the tibia.

_____

For the following axial calcaneal projections with poor positioning, state which anatomic structures are misaligned and how the patient should be repositioned for an optimal projection to be obtained.

Figure 6-25

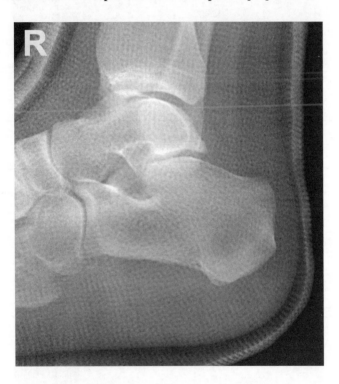

117. Figure 6-25: _____

_____

_____

_____

Chapter **6** **Image Analysis of the Lower Extremity**

Figure 6-26

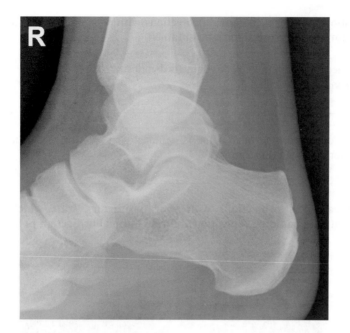

118. Figure 6-26: _____

_____

_____

_____

Figure 6-27

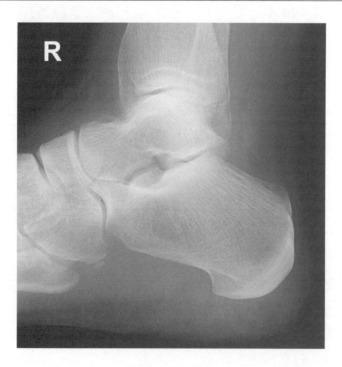

119. Figure 6-27: _____

_____

_____

_____

Ankle: AP Projection

120. Identify the labeled anatomy in Figure 6-28.

Figure 6-28

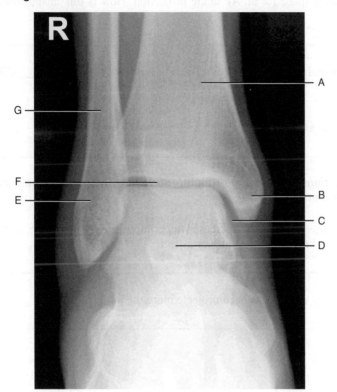

A. _____

B. _____

C. _____

D. _____

E. _____

F. _____

G. _____

121. Complete the statements below referring to AP ankle projection analysis guidelines.

AP Ankle Projection Analysis Guidelines
■ The medial mortise is open, and the tibia superimposes (A) _____ of the distal fibula.
■ The tibiotalar joint space is (B) _____, and the tibia is demonstrated without foreshortening.
■ The (C) _____ is at the center of the exposure field.

122. The ankle joint is located at the same level as what palpable anatomic structure?

_____

123. Is the distal fibula superimposed by the tibia or is the tibia superimposed by the distal fibula on an AP ankle projection?

_____

124. The patient's leg was laterally rotated for an AP ankle projection. How can this mispositioning be identified on an AP ankle projection?

_____

_____

Chapter **6 Image Analysis of the Lower Extremity**

125. How is the patient positioned for an AP ankle projection to obtain an open tibiotalar joint space?

_____

126. The CR was centered proximal to the ankle joint space for an AP ankle projection. How is this mispositioning identified on an AP ankle projection?

_____

127. Accurate CR centering on an AP ankle projection is accomplished by centering a(n) (A) _____ CR to the ankle midline at the level of the (B) _____.

128. Which anatomic structures are included on an AP ankle projection with accurate positioning?

_____

For the following descriptions of AP ankle projections with poor positioning, state how the patient would have been mispositioned for such a projection to be obtained.

129. The medial mortise is obscured, the tibia and talus demonstrate increased superimposition of the fibula, and the posterior aspect of the medial malleolus is situated medial to the anterior aspect.

_____

130. The tibiotalar joint is closed, and the anterior tibial margin has been projected into the joint space.

_____

For the following AP ankle projection with poor positioning, state which anatomic structures are misaligned and how the patient should be repositioned for an optimal projection to be obtained.

Figure 6-29

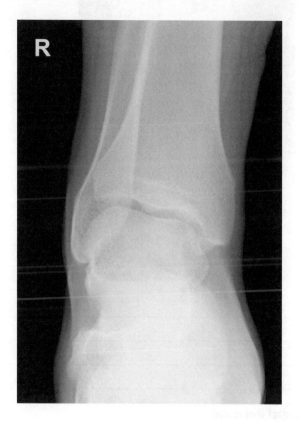

131. Figure 6-29: _____

_____

_____

_____

Figure 6-30

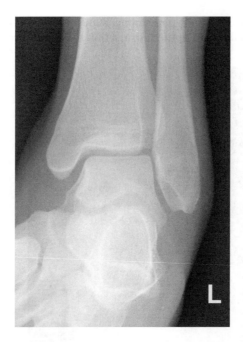

132. Figure 6-30: _____

_____

_____

_____

Ankle: AP Oblique Projection (Medial Rotation)

133. Identify the labeled anatomy in Figure 6-31.

Figure 6-31

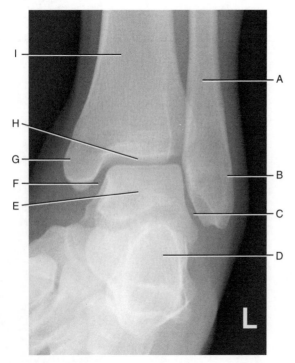

A. _____

B. _____

C. _____

D. _____

E. _____

F. _____

G. _____

H. _____

I. _____

134. Complete the statements below referring to AP oblique ankle projection analysis guidelines.

AP Oblique Ankle Projection Analysis Guidelines
■ Mortise (15–20 degree) oblique: Distal fibula is demonstrated without (A) _____ superimposition, demonstrating an open (B) _____ mortise, and the lateral and medial malleoli are in profile. The tibia superimposes one-fourth of the (C) _____.
■ 45-degree oblique: The fibula is seen without (D) _____ superimposition, and the tarsi sinus is demonstrated.
■ The calcaneus is visualized (E) _____ to the lateral mortise and fibula.
■ The (F) _____ is at the center of the exposure field.

135. Approximately how much ankle obliquity is needed for a mortise AP oblique ankle projection with accurate positioning?

    A. _____

    In which direction is the patient's leg rotated?

    B. _____

136. The intermalleolar line is at what angle with the IR when the patient is accurately positioned for an AP ankle projection?

    _____

137. How is the patient positioned to obtain an open tibiotalar joint space on an AP oblique ankle projection with accurate positioning?

    _____

138. How is the patient positioned to demonstrate the calcaneus distal to the lateral mortise and fibula on an AP oblique ankle projection?

    _____

139. Accurate CR centering on an AP oblique ankle projection is accomplished by centering a(n) (A) _____ CR to the ankle midline at the level of the (B) _____.

140. Which anatomic structures are included on an AP ankle projection with accurate positioning?

    _____

For the following descriptions of AP oblique ankle projections with poor positioning, state how the patient would have been mispositioned for such a projection to be obtained.

141. Mortise oblique: The lateral and medial mortises are closed, and the tarsal sinus is demonstrated.

    _____

142. 45-degree oblique: The lateral and medial mortises are closed, the fibula is demonstrated without tibial superimposition, and the tarsal sinus is demonstrated.

    _____

143. Mortise oblique: The tibiotalar joint space is expanded, the anterior tibial margin is projected superior to the posterior margin, and the tibial articulating surface is demonstrated.

_____

144. 45-degree oblique: The calcaneus is obscuring the distal aspect of the lateral mortise and the distal fibula.

_____

For the following AP oblique ankle projections with poor positioning, state which anatomic structures are misaligned and how the patient should be repositioned for an optimal projection to be obtained.

Figure 6-32

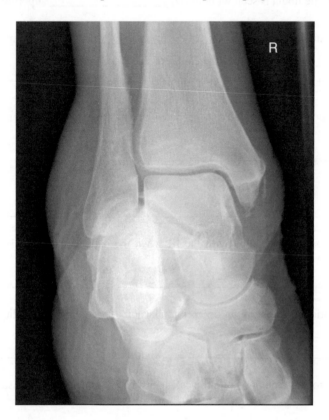

145. Figure 6-32, mortise oblique: _____

_____

_____

_____

Figure 6-33

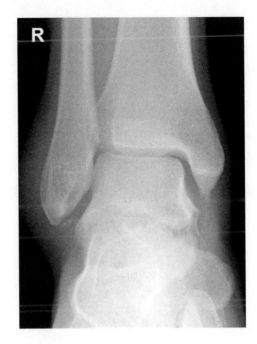

146. Figure 6-33, mortise oblique: _____

_____

_____

_____

Figure 6-34

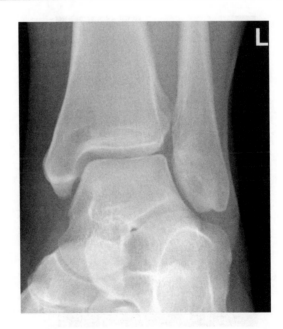

147. Figure 6-34, 45-degree oblique: _____

_____

_____

_____

Figure 6-35

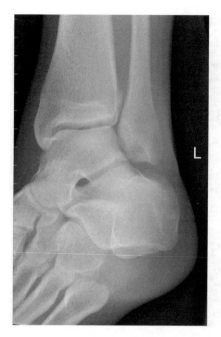

148. Figure 6-35, 45-degree oblique: _____

_____

_____

_____

Figure 6-36

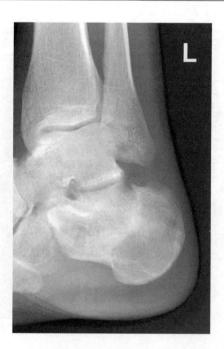

149. Figure 6-36, 45-degree oblique: _____

_____

_____

_____

Figure 6-37

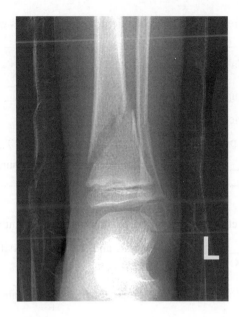

150. Figure 6-37, trauma, 45-degree oblique: _____

_____

_____

_____

Ankle: Lateral Projection (Mediolateral)

151. Identify the labeled anatomy in Figure 6-38.

Figure 6-38

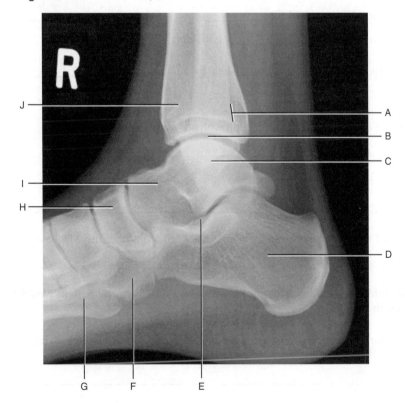

A. _____

B. _____

C. _____

D. _____

E. _____

F. _____

G. _____

H. _____

I. _____

J. _____

152. Complete the statements below referring to lateral ankle projection analysis guidelines.

┌───┐
│ **Lateral Ankle Projection Analysis Guidelines**   │
│   │
│ ■ The talar domes are superimposed, the tibiotalar joint is (A) _____, and the distal fibula is │
│   superimposed by the posterior half of the (B) _____.   │
│ ■ The long axis of the foot is positioned at a 90-degree angle with the (C) _____. │
│ ■ The (D) _____ is at the center of the exposure field.   │
└───┘

153. To obtain a lateral ankle projection with accurate positioning, the patient's leg is extended, the lower leg is

   positioned (A) _____ to the IR, and the foot is dorsiflexed with its (B) _____
   surface aligned parallel to the IR.

154. Accurate lower leg positioning for a lateral ankle projection ensures accurate _____ alignment of the
   talar domes.

155. If the proximal lower leg is positioned farther from the imaging table than the distal tibia for a lateral ankle projec-

   tion, the (A) _____ dome is demonstrated (B) _____ to the (C) _____

   talar dome, and the longitudinal foot arch appears (D) _____ on the resulting projection.

156. Accurate lateral foot surface positioning for a lateral ankle projection ensures proper (A) _____

   and (B) _____ alignment of the talar domes.

157. If the forefoot is positioned too close to the IR and the calcaneus is raised off the IR for a lateral ankle projection,

   the (A) _____ talar domes are demonstrated (B) _____ to the (C) _____ talar

   dome, and the fibula is demonstrated too far (D) _____ on the tibia.

158. Accurate CR centering on a lateral ankle projection is accomplished by centering a(n) (A) _____

   CR to the (B) _____.

159. Which anatomic structures are included on a lateral ankle projection with accurate positioning?

   _____

160. What is a Jones fracture?

   _____

161. Why should the transversely collimated field remain open to include 1 inch (2.5 cm) of the fifth MT base?

   _____

For the following descriptions of lateral ankle projections with poor positioning, state how the patient would have been mispositioned for such a projection to be obtained.

162. Average longitudinal arch: The tibiotalar joint space is obscured, one talar dome is demonstrated proximal to the
   other dome, and more than 0.5 inch (1.25 cm) of the cuboid appears posterior to the navicular.

   _____

163. The tibiotalar joint is obscured, one talar dome is demonstrated anterior to the other dome, and the fibula is demonstrated too anterior on the tibia.

___

For the following lateral ankle projections with poor positioning, state which anatomic structures are misaligned and how the patient should be repositioned for an optimal projection to be obtained.

Figure 6-39

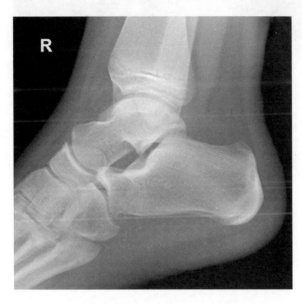

164. Figure 6-39: _____

_____

_____

_____

Figure 6-40

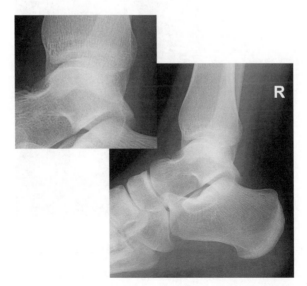

165. Figure 6-40: _____

_____

_____

_____

Figure 6-41

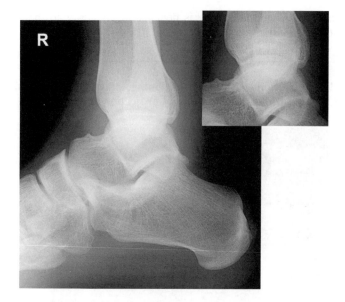

166. Figure 6-41: _____

_____

_____

_____

Figure 6-42

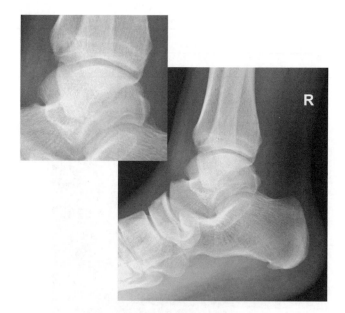

167. Figure 6-42, trauma, lateromedial projection: _____

_____

_____

_____

Figure 6-43

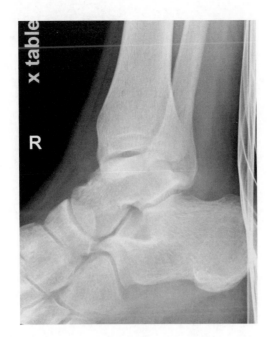

168. Figure 6-43, trauma, lateromedial projection: _____

_____

_____

_____

Figure 6-44

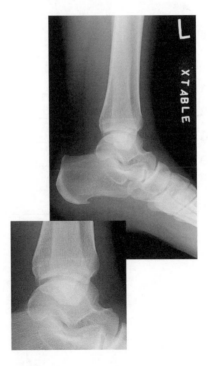

169. Figure 6-44, trauma, lateromedial projection: _____

_____

_____

_____

Figure 6-45

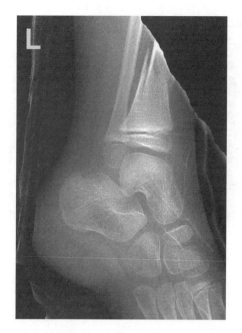

170. Figure 6-45, trauma, lateromedial projection: _____

_____

_____

_____

Lower Leg: AP Projection

171. Identify the labeled anatomy in Figure 6-46.

Figure 6-46

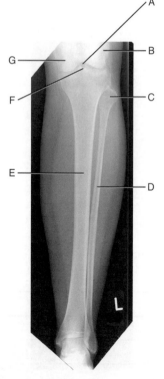

A. _____

B. _____

C. _____

D. _____

E. _____

F. _____

G. _____

172. Complete the statements below referring to AP lower leg projection analysis guidelines.

AP Lower Leg Projection Analysis Guidelines
■ The tibia superimposes about (A) _____ of the fibular head and about (B) _____ of the distal tibia.
■ The fibular midshaft is (C) _____ of tibial superimposition.
■ The knee and tibiotalar joint spaces are (D) _____.
■ The (E) _____ is at the center of the exposure field.

173. How should the lower leg be positioned with respect to the x-ray tube to take advantage of the anode-heel effect?

_____

174. Describe how the tibia and fibula on an AP lower leg projection are misaligned at the knee and ankle if the leg is internally rotated.

   A. Knee: _____

   B. Ankle: _____

175. A patient from the emergency department is unable to position the ankle and knee in an AP projection simultaneously for an AP lower leg projection. If the area of interest is closer to the knee joint, how should the leg be positioned for the projection?

_____

176. Are the femorotibial and tibiotalar joint spaces closed on an AP lower leg projection with accurate positioning?

   A. _____ (Yes/No)

   B. Explain how the divergence of the x-ray beam used to record these two joints affects their openness.

177. Why is it necessary for the IR to extend at least 1 inch (2.5 cm) beyond the ankle and knee joints when the lower leg is positioned in an AP projection?

_____

178. The ankle joint is located at the level of the (A) _____, and the knee joint is located 1 inch (2.5 cm)

   (B) _____ to the (C) _____.

179. The _____ is centered to the collimated field on an AP lower leg projection with accurate positioning.

180. Which anatomic structures are included on an AP lower leg projection with accurate positioning?

_____

For the following descriptions of AP lower leg projections with poor positioning, state how the patient would have been mispositioned for such a projection to be obtained.

181. The medial mortise is closed, and the tibia and talus demonstrate excessive fibular superimposition.

_____

182. The distal fibula is free of talar superimposition, and the proximal fibula is free of tibial superimposition.

For the following AP lower leg projection with poor positioning, state which anatomic structures are misaligned and how the patient should be repositioned for an optimal projection to be obtained.

Figure 6-47

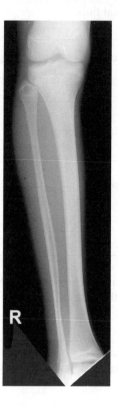

183. Figure 6-47: _____

_____

_____

_____

Lower Leg: Lateral Projection (Mediolateral)

184. Identify the labeled anatomy in Figure 6-48.

Figure 6-48

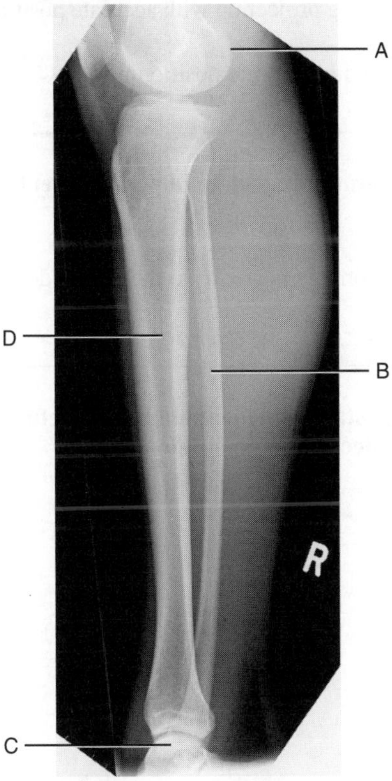

A. _____

B. _____

C. _____

D. _____

185. Complete the statements below referring to lateral lower leg projection analysis guidelines.

Lateral Lower Leg Projection Analysis Guidelines
■ The tibia superimposes about (A) _____ of the fibular head, and the (B) _____ aspects of the distal tibia and fibula are aligned.
■ The fibular (C) _____ is free of tibial superimposition.
■ The (D) _____ is at the center of the exposure field.

186. Describe the anatomic relationship of the tibia and fibula at the knee, midshaft, and ankle on a lateral lower leg projection with accurate positioning.

A. Knee: _____

B. Midshaft: _____

C. Ankle: _____

187. How does the relationship between the tibia and fibula at the knee and ankle described in the previous question change if the patient's medial femoral epicondyle is rotated anterior to the lateral epicondyle for the projection?

A. Knee: _____

B. Ankle: _____

281

188. To ensure that the ankle and knee joints are included on a lateral lower leg projection, how far should the IR and longitudinally collimated field extend beyond them?

_____

189. The _____ is centered to the collimated field on a lateral lower leg projection with accurate positioning.

190. Which anatomic structures are included on a lateral lower leg projection with accurate positioning?

_____

For the following descriptions of lateral lower leg projections with poor positioning, state how the patient would have been mispositioned for such a projection to be obtained.

191. The distal fibula is situated too far anterior on the tibia, the medial talar dome is posterior to the lateral dome, and the fibular head and midshaft are superimposed by the tibia.

_____

For the following lateral lower leg projections with poor positioning, state which anatomic structures are misaligned and how the patient should be repositioned for an optimal projection to be obtained.

Figure 6-49

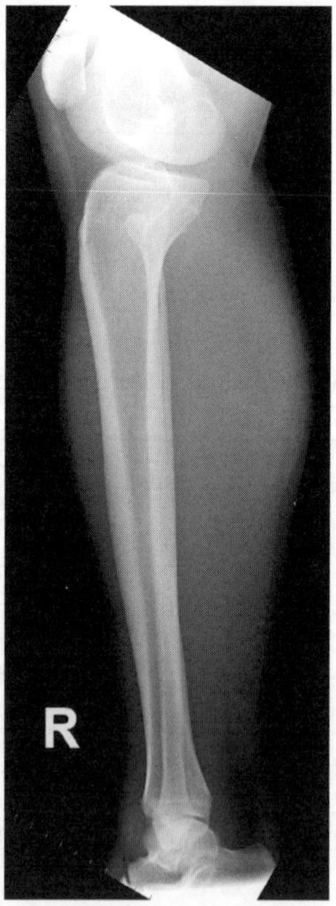

192. Figure 6-49: _____

_____

_____

_____

Figure 6-50

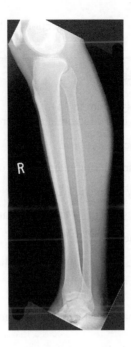

193. Figure 6-50: _____

_____

_____

_____

Knee: AP Projection

194. Identify the labeled anatomy in Figure 6-51.

Figure 6-51

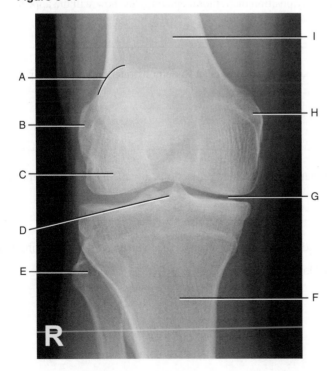

A. _____

B. _____

C. _____

D. _____

E. _____

F. _____

G. _____

H. _____

I. _____

195. Complete the statements below referring to AP knee projection analysis guidelines.

AP Knee Projection Analysis Guidelines

- The medial and lateral femoral epicondyles are in (A) _____, the femoral condyles are symmetrical, the intercondylar eminence is centered within the intercondylar fossa, and the tibia is superimposed over (B) _____ of the fibular head.

- The femorotibial joint space is open, the anterior and posterior distal tibial margins are aligned, and the fibular head is demonstrated approximately 0.5 inch (1.25 cm) distal to the (C) _____.

- The patella lies just (D) _____ to the patellar surface of the femur and is situated slightly (E) _____ to the knee midline.

- The (F) _____ is at the center of the exposure field.

---

196. A grid is used for a knee projection if the patient's knee measures more than _____ cm.

197. An AP knee projection is obtained by placing the patient supine with the knee (A) _____ and leg (B) _____ rotated until the femoral epicondyles are placed at (C) _____ from the IR.

198. Is the proximal tibia superimposed over the proximal fibula or is the proximal fibula superimposed over the proximal tibia when the knee is in an AP projection?

_____

199. If the knee is rotated from an AP projection, will the femoral condyle positioned closer to or farther away from the IR appear larger on the resulting projection?

200. If the patient's leg is not internally rotated to accurately position the femoral epicondyles, how will the appearances of the femoral condyles and the alignment of the tibia and fibula change?

_____

201. How is the CR aligned with the femorotibial joint space and tibial plateau to demonstrate them as open spaces on an AP knee projection?

202. Describe the slope of the tibial plateau.

_____

203. Why is it necessary to vary the degree of CR angulation for AP knee projections in patients with different upper thigh and buttock thicknesses?

_____

204. Should the patient's abdominal thickness be included in the anterior superior iliac spine (ASIS)-to-imaging table measurement obtained for a patient undergoing AP knee imaging? _____ (Yes/No)

205. What CR angulation is used when obtaining an AP knee projection in a patient with a large (24 cm) ASIS-to-imaging table measurement?

A. _____

When imaging a patient with a small (18 cm) ASIS-to-imaging table measurement?

B. _____

206. If the wrong CR angle is used for an AP knee projection, the shape of the fibular head and its proximity to the tibial plateau change from that demonstrated on an AP knee projection in which an accurate CR angle was used. For each situation that follows, state the change that occurs.

A. CR angled too cephalically: _____

B. CR angled too caudally: _____

207. Which knee compartment on an AP knee projection is the narrower when a valgus deformity is present?

A. _____

When a varus deformity is present?

B. _____

208. What deformity is demonstrated in Figure 6-52?

Figure 6-52

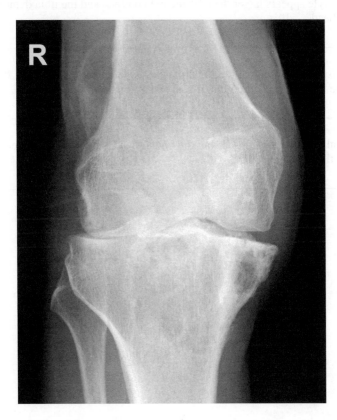

209. An AP knee projection is requested for a patient who is unable to fully extend the knee. The technologist angled the CR until it was perpendicular to the anterior surface of the lower leg and obtained a 10-degree cephalic angle. How is this angle adjusted to align the CR parallel with the tibial plateau and obtain an open femorotibial joint?

210. When the knee is flexed, the patella shifts (A) _____ (proximally/distally) and (B) _____ (medially/laterally) onto the patellar surface of the femur and then (C) _____ (medially/laterally) onto the intercondylar fossa.

211. Accurate CR centering on an AP knee projection is accomplished by centering the CR (A) _____ inch(es) (B) _____ to the palpable (C) _____.

212. Which anatomic structures are included on an AP knee projection with accurate positioning?

_____

For the following descriptions of AP knee projections with poor positioning, state how the patient or CR would have been mispositioned for such a projection to be obtained.

213. The medial femoral condyle appears larger than the lateral condyle, and the head, neck, and shaft of the fibula are almost entirely superimposed by the tibia.

_____

214. The lateral femoral condyle appears larger than the medial condyle, and the tibia demonstrates very little superimposition of the fibular head.

_____

215. The femorotibial joint space is obscured, the tibial plateau is demonstrated, and the fibular head is foreshortened and demonstrated more than 0.5 inch (1.25 cm) distal to the tibial plateau.

_____

216. The medial femorotibial joint space is closed, and the fibular head is elongated and demonstrated less than 0.5 inch (1.25 cm) distal to the tibial plateau.

_____

For the following AP knee projections with poor positioning, state which anatomic structures are misaligned and how the patient should be repositioned for an optimal projection to be obtained.

Figure 6-53

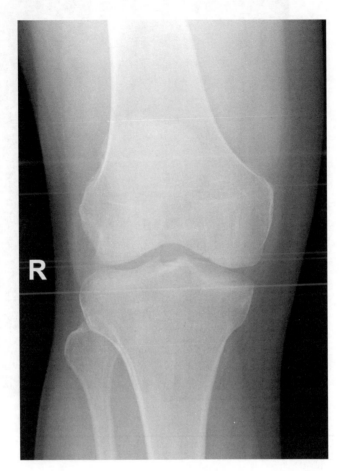

217. Figure 6-53: _____

_____

_____

_____

Figure 6-54

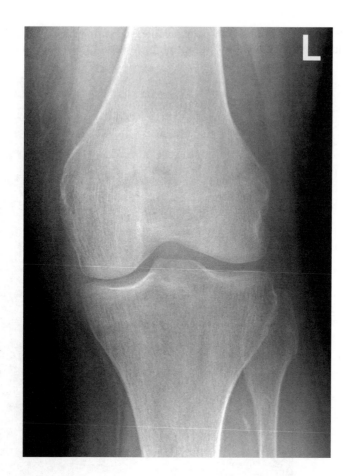

218. Figure 6-54: _____

_____

_____

_____

Figure 6-55

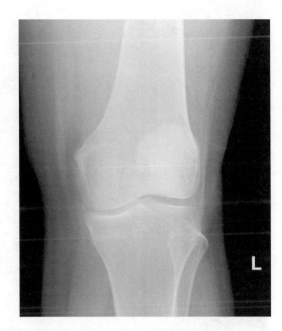

219. Figure 6-55: _____

_____

_____

_____

Figure 6-56

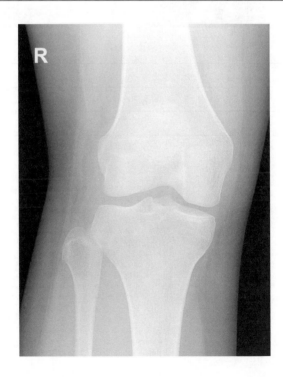

220. Figure 6-56: _____

_____

_____

_____

Figure 6-57

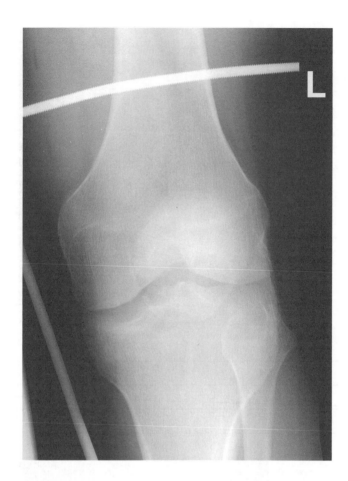

221. Figure 6-57, trauma: _____

_____

_____

_____

Figure 6-58

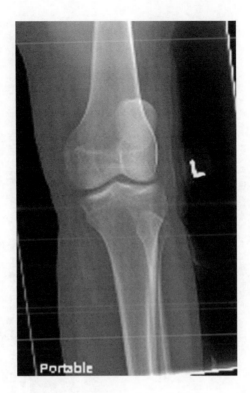

222. Figure 6-58, trauma: _____

_____

_____

_____

Figure 6-59

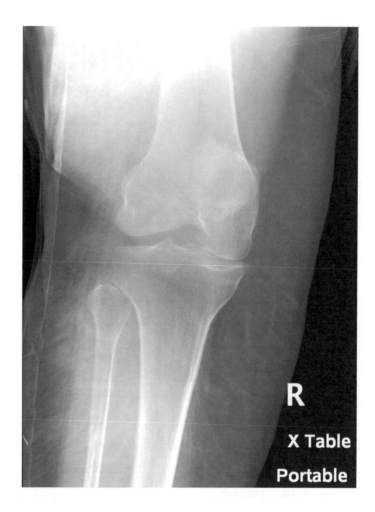

R

X Table

Portable

223. Figure 6-59, trauma; this was taken cross-table: _____

_____

_____

_____

Knee: AP Oblique Projection (Medial and Lateral Rotation)

224. Identify the labeled anatomy in Figure 6-60.

Figure 6-60

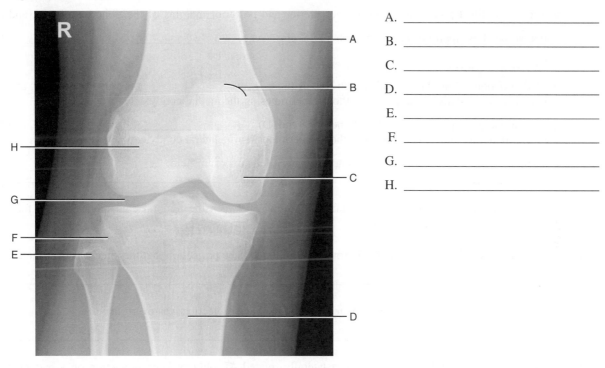

A. _____

B. _____

C. _____

D. _____

E. _____

F. _____

G. _____

H. _____

225. Identify the labeled anatomy in Figure 6-61.

Figure 6-61

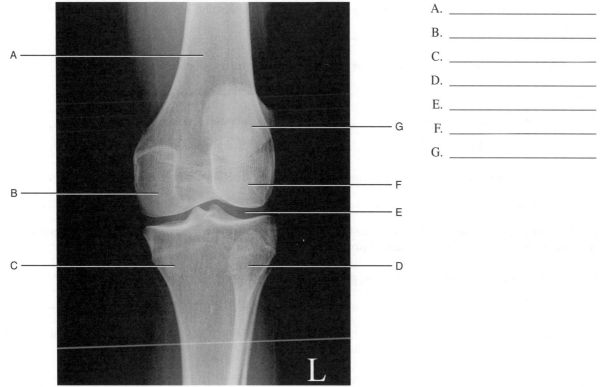

A. _____

B. _____

C. _____

D. _____

E. _____

F. _____

G. _____

226. Complete the statements below referring to AP oblique knee projection analysis guidelines.

> **AP Oblique Knee Projection Analysis Guidelines**
>
> - The femorotibial joint space is open, the anterior and posterior margins of the tibia are aligned, and the fibular head is approximately 0.5 inch (1.25 cm) (A) _____ to the (B) _____ .
> - Medial oblique: The fibular head is seen free of (C) _____ superimposition, and the lateral femoral condyle is in profile without superimposing the medial condyle.
> - Lateral oblique: The fibular head is aligned with the (D) _____ edge of the tibia, and the medial femoral condyle is in profile without superimposing the lateral condyle.
> - The (E) _____ is at the center of the exposure field.

227. For AP oblique knee projections, an imaginary line drawn between the femoral epicondyles should form a(n) _____-degree angle with the IR.

228. How can one determine from an internally rotated AP oblique knee projection that the knee was overrotated?

_____

229. How can one determine if an externally rotated AP oblique knee projection was overrotated?

_____

230. What degree of CR angulation is used for a laterally rotated AP oblique knee projection on a patient whose ASIS-to-imaging table measurement is 12 cm?

A. _____

Why is it common to need a cephalic angle for the medially (internally) AP oblique knee projection?

B. _____

Why is it common to need a caudal angle for the lateral (externally) AP oblique knee projection?

C. _____

231. The CR is centered to the (A) _____ at a level (B) _____inch(es) (C) _____ to the palpable (D)_____ for AP oblique knee projections.

232. Which anatomic structures are included on an oblique knee projection with accurate positioning?

_____

For the following descriptions of AP oblique knee projections with poor positioning, state how the patient or CR would have been mispositioned for such a projection to be obtained.

233. On an internally rotated knee projection, the tibia is partially superimposed over the fibular head.

_____

234. On an externally rotated knee projection, the lateral femoral condyle is superimposed over the medial condyle, and the fibula is located in the center of the tibia.

_____

294

235. On an externally rotated knee projection, the fibula is not entirely superimposed by the tibia.

_____

236. On an internally rotated knee projection, the femorotibial joint space is obscured, and the fibular head is foreshortened and demonstrated more than 0.5 inch (1.25 cm) distal to the tibial plateau.

_____

For the following AP oblique knee projections with poor positioning, state which anatomic structures are misaligned and how the patient should be repositioned for an optimal projection to be obtained.

Figure 6-62

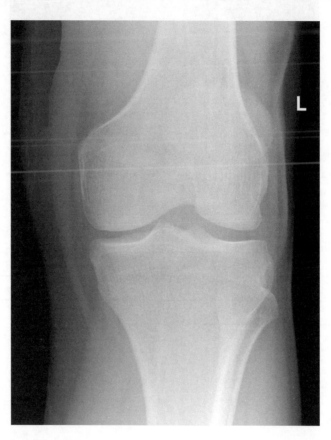

237. Figure 6-62 lateral oblique: _____

_____

_____

_____

Figure 6-63

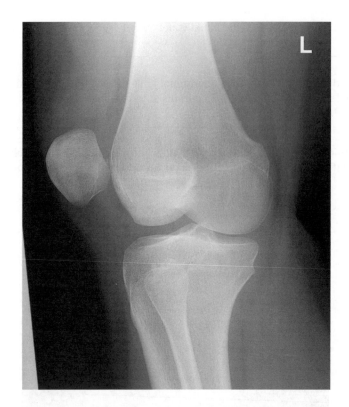

238. Figure 6-63, lateral oblique: _____

_____

_____

_____

Figure 6-64

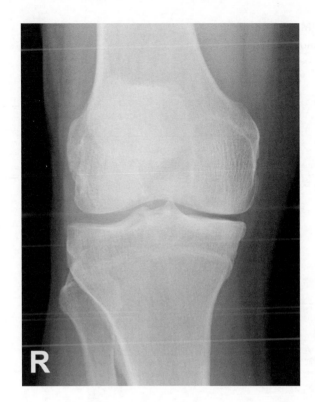

239. Figure 6-64, medial oblique: _____

_____

_____

_____

Knee: Lateral Projection (Mediolateral)

240. Identify the labeled anatomy in Figure 6-65.

Figure 6-65

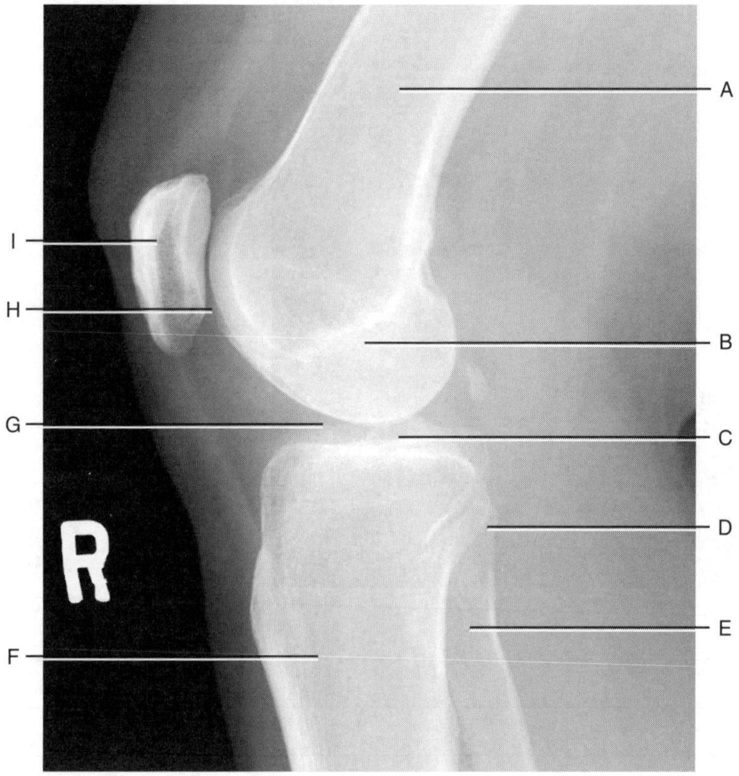

A. _____

B. _____

C. _____

D. _____

E. _____

F. _____

G. _____

H. _____

I. _____

241. Complete the statements below referring to lateral knee projection analysis guidelines.

Lateral Knee Projection Analysis Guidelines
■ Contrast and density are adequate to demonstrate the (A) _____ fat pad.
■ The patella is situated (B) _____ to the patellar surface of the femur, and the patellofemoral joint is open.
■ The distal articulating surfaces of the medial and lateral (C) _____ are aligned, and the knee joint space is open.
■ The anterior and posterior surfaces of the medial and lateral femoral condyles are aligned, and the tibia superimposes one-half of the (D) _____.
■ The (E) _____ is at the center of the exposure field.

242. Why can a joint effusion diagnosis be made when evaluating a lateral knee projection if the knee is flexed less than 20 degrees but becomes difficult to make when the knee is flexed more than 20 degrees?

_____

_____

243. When a patient is erect, the distal femoral condylar surfaces are aligned (A) _____ to the floor, and the femoral shaft inclines (B) _____ up to (C) _____ degrees. A patient who demonstrates the greatest femoral inclination will have a (D) _____ (wide/narrow) pelvis and (E) _____ (long/short) femoral shaft length.

244. When the average patient is placed in a recumbent lateral position for a lateral knee projection, the femoral shaft inclination displayed in the erect position is reduced, causing the (A) _____ condyle to be projected (B) _____ to the (C) _____ condyle.

245. To obtain superimposed distal femoral condylar surfaces when imaging the average patient for a lateral knee projection, a(n) (A) _____-degree cephalic CR angulation is used to shift the (B) _____ condyle anteriorly and proximally. The CR angulation is (C) _____ (increased/reduced) when imaging a patient with a narrow pelvis and long femora.

246. State two methods of distinguishing the medial femoral condyle from the lateral femoral condyle on a lateral knee projection with poor positioning.

   A. _____

   B. _____

247. When is it necessary to use a cephalic CR angulation for a cross-table lateral knee projection in a patient in a supine position?

   _____

   _____

248. What is the relationship between the tibia and the fibular head on a lateral knee projection with accurate positioning if superimposed condyles were obtained by aligning the femoral epicondyles perpendicular to the IR and directing the CR across the femur to project the medial condyle anteriorly and proximally?

   A. _____

   How will this relationship change if superimposed condyles are obtained by rolling the patient's patella approximately 0.25 inch (0.6 cm) closer to the IR and directing the CR toward the femur so it only moves the medial condyle proximally?

   B. _____

249. Why is the medial condyle shifted more than the lateral condyle when the degree of CR angulation is adjusted?

   _____

250. If the medial condyle is demonstrated anterior to the lateral condyle on a lateral knee projection with poor positioning, what will the tibia and fibular relationship be?

   _____

251. If the lateral condyle is demonstrated anterior to the medial condyle on a lateral knee projection with poor positioning, what will the tibia and fibular relationship be?

   _____

252. Accurate CR centering on a lateral knee projection is accomplished by centering the CR to the midline of the knee at a level (A) _____ inch(es) (B) _____ to the palpable (C) _____.

299

253. Which anatomic structures are included on a lateral knee projection with accurate positioning?

_____

For the following descriptions of lateral knee projections with poor positioning, state how the patient or CR would have been mispositioned for such a projection to be obtained.

254. The patient's patella is in contact with the patellar surface of the femur, and the suprapatellar fat pads are obscured.

_____

255. The distal articulating surfaces of the femoral condyles are demonstrated without superimposition. The condyle that has the adductor tubercle attached to it is demonstrated approximately 0.25 inch (0.6 cm) distal to the other condyle.

_____

256. The distal articulating surfaces of the femoral condyles are demonstrated without superimposition. The condyle that has the flattest distal surface is demonstrated approximately 0.5 inch (1.25 cm) distal to the other condyle.

_____

257. The anterior and posterior aspects of the femoral condyles are demonstrated without superimposition. The medial condyle is demonstrated posteriorly.

_____

258. The anterior and posterior aspects of the femoral condyles are demonstrated without superimposition. The medial condyle is demonstrated anteriorly.

_____

For the following lateral knee projections with poor positioning, state which anatomic structures are misaligned and how the patient should be repositioned for an optimal projection to be obtained.

Figure 6-66

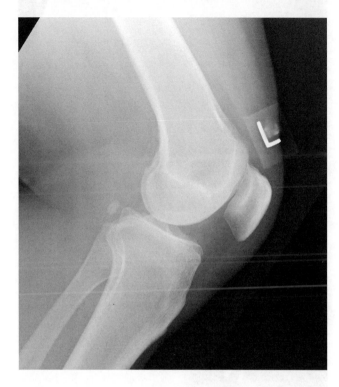

259. Figure 6-66: _____

_____

_____

_____

Figure 6-67

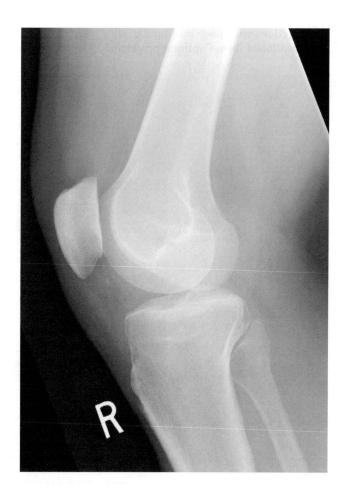

260. Figure 6-67: _____

_____

_____

_____

Figure 6-68

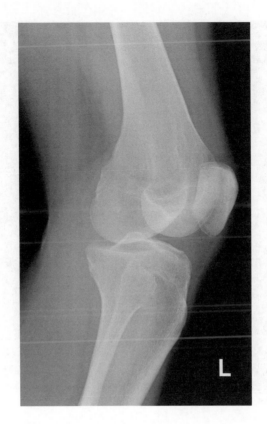

261. Figure 6-68: _____

_____

_____

_____

Figure 6-69

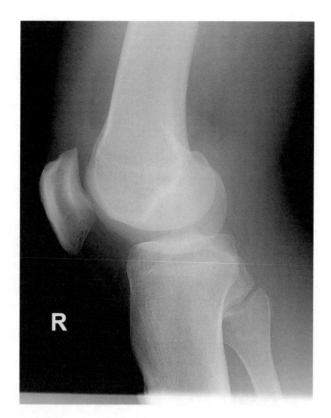

262. Figure 6-69: _____

_____

_____

_____

Figure 6-70

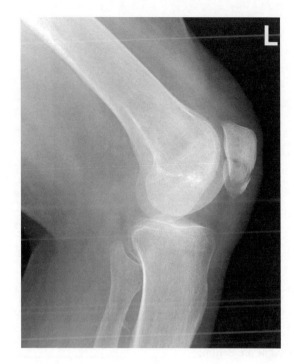

263. Figure 6-70, trauma, mediolateral projection: _____

_____

_____

_____

Figure 6-71

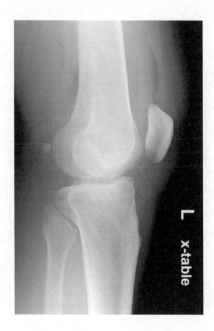

264. Figure 6-71, trauma, lateromedial projection: _____

_____

_____

_____

Figure 6-72

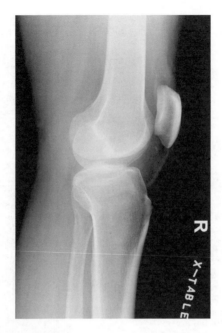

265. Figure 6-72, trauma, lateromedial projection: _____

_____

_____

_____

Figure 6-73

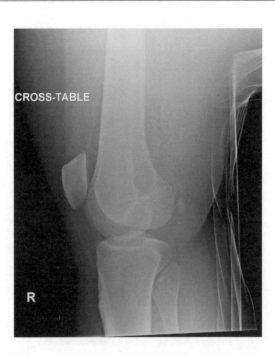

266. Figure 6-73, trauma, lateromedial projection: _____

_____

_____

_____

Intercondylar Fossa: PA Axial Projection (Holmblad Method)

267. Identify the labeled anatomy in Figure 6-74.

Figure 6-74

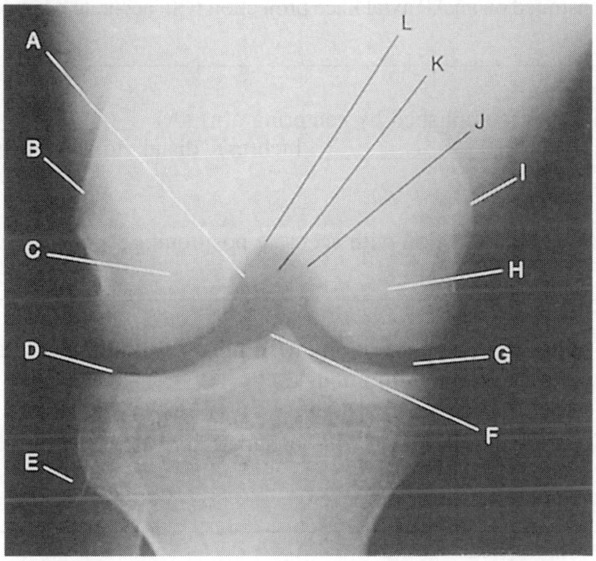

A. _____

B. _____

C. _____

D. _____

E. _____

F. _____

G. _____

H. _____

I. _____

J. _____

K. _____

L. _____

268. Complete the statements below referring to PA axial (Holmblad method) knee projection analysis guidelines.

PA Axial (Holmblad Method) Knee Projection Analysis Guidelines

■ The medial and lateral surfaces of the intercondylar fossa and the femoral epicondyles are in profile, and

(A) _____ of the fibular head superimposes the proximal tibia.

■ The proximal surface of the intercondylar fossa is in (B) _____, and the patellar apex

is demonstrated (C) _____ to the intercondylar fossa.

■ The knee joint space is (D) _____, and the tibial plateau and intercondylar eminence and
the tubercles are in profile. The fibular head is demonstrated approximately 0.25 inch (0.6 cm)

(E) _____ to the tibial plateau.

■ The (F) _____ is at the center of the exposure field.

---

269. How are the femur and foot positioned to demonstrate superimposed medial and lateral intercondylar fossa surfaces on a PA axial knee projection?

A. Femur: _____

B. Foot: _____

270. In which direction does the patella move when the patient is positioned for a PA axial knee projection and the heel is rotated as indicated below?

A. Medially: _____

B. Laterally: _____

271. To superimpose the proximal surfaces of the intercondylar fossa in the PA axial knee position, position the patient's femur at (A) _____ degrees from vertical or (B) _____ degrees from the imaging table.

272. If the knee is flexed more than needed to superimpose the proximal surfaces of the intercondylar fossa, is the patella demonstrated proximally or distally to where it is demonstrated on an AP axial knee projection with accurate positioning?

_____

273. Accurate CR centering on a PA axial knee projection is accomplished by centering a(n) (A) _____ CR to the midline of the knee at a level (B) _____ inch(es) distal to the palpable (C) _____.

274. Which anatomic structures are included on a PA axial knee projection with accurate positioning?

_____

For the following descriptions of PA axial (Holmblad method) knee projections with poor positioning, state how the patient would have been mispositioned for such a projection to be obtained.

275. The medial and lateral aspects of the intercondylar fossa are demonstrated without superimposition, and the patella is situated laterally.

_____

276. The medial and lateral aspects of the intercondylar fossa are demonstrated without superimposition, the patella is situated medially, and the tibia is demonstrated without fibular head superimposition.

_____

277. The proximal surfaces of the intercondylar fossa are demonstrated without superimposition, and the patella is positioned within the intercondylar fossa.

_____

278. The proximal surfaces of the intercondylar fossa are demonstrated without superimposition, and the patella is positioned too far proximal to the intercondylar fossa.

_____

279. PA Axial projection (weight-bearing bilateral flexed): demonstrates the posterior margin of the proximal intercondylar fossa at a distance less than 0.25 inch and the patellar apex is next to the intercondylar fossa.

_____

For the following PA axial (Holmblad method) knee projections with poor positioning, state which anatomic structures are misaligned and how the patient should be repositioned for an optimal projection to be obtained.

Figure 6-75

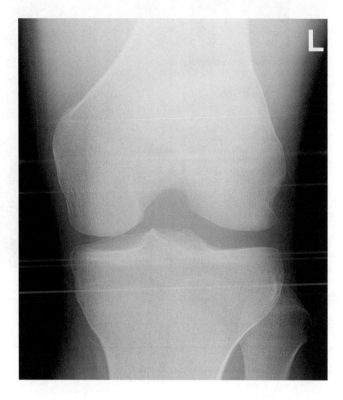

280. Figure 6-75: _____

_____

_____

_____

Figure 6-76

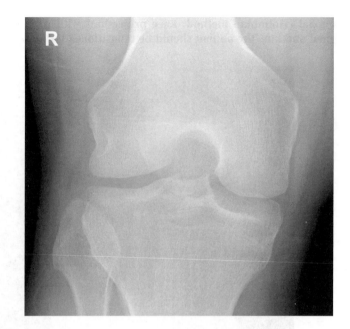

281. Figure 6-76: _____
_____
_____
_____

Figure 6-77

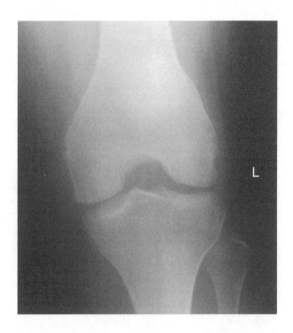

282. Figure 6-77: _____
_____
_____
_____

310

Intercondylar Fossa: AP Axial Projection (Béclere Method)

283. Identify the labeled anatomy in Figure 6-78.

Figure 6-78

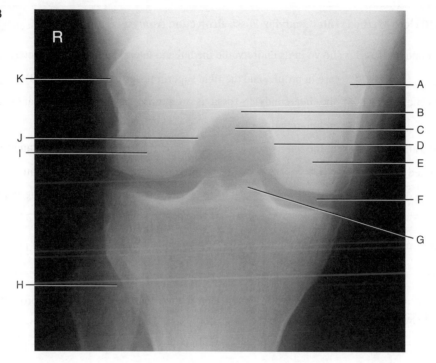

A. _____

B. _____

C. _____

D. _____

E. _____

F. _____

G. _____

H. _____

I. _____

J. _____

K. _____

284. Complete the statements below referring to AP axial (Béclere method) intercondylar fossa projection analysis guidelines.

AP Axial (Béclere Method) Intercondylar Fossa Projection Analysis Guidelines
■ The intercondylar fossa is shown in its entirety, the medial and lateral surfaces of the intercondylar fossa and the (A) _____ are in profile, and the tibia superimposes one-half of the (B) _____. ■ The proximal surface of the intercondylar fossa is in profile, and the patellar apex is demonstrated (C) _____ to the intercondylar fossa. ■ The knee joint space is open, the intercondylar eminence and tubercles are in profile, and the fibular head is demonstrated approximately (D) _____ inch(es) distal to the tibial plateau. ■ The (E) _____ is at the center of the exposure field.

285. How is the knee positioned to superimpose the medial and lateral surfaces on the PA axial projection?

_____

286. How are the CR and the patient positioned to obtain a projection that demonstrates the proximal surfaces of the intercondylar fossa in profile?

A. CR: _____

B. Patient: _____

287. For an open knee joint space and demonstration of the intercondylar eminence and tubercles in profile, the

(A) _____ and (B) _____ must be aligned parallel with each other.

288. Accurate CR centering on an AP axial projection is accomplished by first positioning the CR (A) _____ with the anterior lower leg surface; then (B) _____ the obtained angulation by 5 degrees and center the CR 1 inch (2.5 cm) distal to the (C) _____.

289. Which anatomic structures are included on an AP axial knee projection with accurate positioning?

_____

For the following descriptions of AP axial (Béclere method) knee projections with poor positioning, state how the patient would have been mispositioned for such a projection to be obtained.

290. The medial and lateral aspects of the intercondylar fossa are not superimposed, the lateral femoral condyle is larger than the medial condyle, and the fibular head demonstrates decreased tibial superimposition.

_____

291. The medial and lateral aspects of the intercondylar fossa are not superimposed, the medial femoral condyle is larger than the lateral condyle, and the fibular head demonstrates increased tibial superimposition.

_____

292. The proximal surfaces of the intercondylar fossa are not superimposed, and the patellar apex is demonstrated within the intercondylar fossa.

_____

293. The proximal surfaces of the intercondylar fossa are not superimposed, and the patellar apex is demonstrated proximal to the intercondylar fossa.

_____

294. The knee joint space is closed, and the fibular head is shown less than 0.5 inch (1.25 cm) distal to the tibial plateau.

_____

295. The knee joint space is closed, and the fibular head is shown more than 0.5 inch (1.25 cm) distal to the tibial plateau.

_____

For the following AP axial (Béclere method) knee projections with poor positioning, state which anatomic structures are misaligned and how the patient should be repositioned for an optimal projection to be obtained.

Figure 6-79

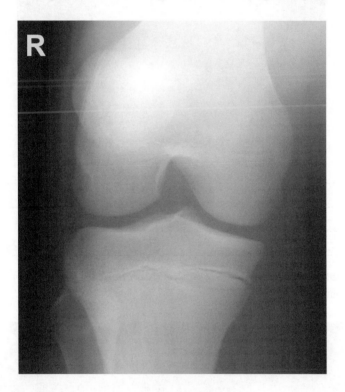

296. Figure 6-79: _____

_____

_____

_____

Chapter **6 Image Analysis of the Lower Extremity**

Figure 6-80

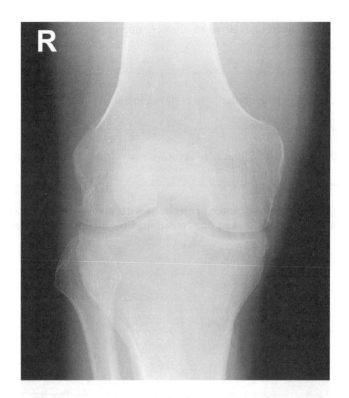

297. Figure 6-80: _____

_____

_____

_____

Patella and Patellofemoral Joint: Tangential Projection (Merchant Method)

298. Identify the labeled anatomy in Figure 6-81.

Figure 6-81

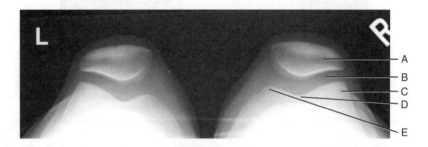

A. _____

B. _____

C. _____

D. _____

E. _____

299. Complete the statements below referring to tangential (Merchant method) patella projection analysis guidelines.

Tangential (Merchant Method) Patella and Patellofemoral Joint Projection Analysis Guidelines
■ The patellae, anterior femoral condyles, and intercondylar sulci are seen superiorly, and the (A) _____ femoral condyle demonstrates slightly more height than the (B) _____ condyle.
■ The patellofemoral joint spaces are (C) _____ with no superimposition of the patellae or tibial tuberosities.
■ A point midway between the (D) _____ is at the center of the exposure field.

300. How are the legs positioned to prevent rotation on a tangential knee projection?

_____

301. How do the positions of the patellae and femoral condyles change when the knees are in external rotation for a tangential knee projection?

A. Patellae: _____

B. Femoral condyles: _____

302. The tangential knee projection is most often obtained to demonstrate which patient condition?

A. _____

How is this condition demonstrated on a tangential knee projection with accurate positioning?

B. _____

How can one distinguish this condition from rotation on a tangential knee projection?

C. _____

303. Why is it important for the patient to relax the quadriceps femoris muscles for the tangential knee projection?

_____

304. How are the femurs positioned to obtain a tangential knee projection with accurate positioning?

_____

305. Where are the posterior knee curves positioned with respect to the axial viewer for a tangential knee projection with accurate positioning?

_____

306. How is the positioning setup for a tangential knee projection adjusted when imaging a patient with large posterior calves?

A. _____

If this positioning setup is not changed, what anatomic misalignment appears on the resulting projection?

B. _____

315

307. What are the standard direction and degree of CR angulation used for the tangential knee projection?

_____

308. What is the sum of the CR angle and the angle of the axial viewer for all tangential knee projections?

_____

309. Which anatomic structures are included on a tangential knee projection with accurate positioning?

_____

For the following descriptions of tangential knee projections with poor positioning, state how the patient would have been mispositioned for such a projection to be obtained.

310. The patellae are demonstrated directly above the intercondylar sulci and rotated laterally. The medial femoral condyles demonstrate more height than the lateral condyles.

_____

311. Soft tissue from the patient's anterior thighs has been projected onto the patellae and patellofemoral joint spaces.

_____

312. The patellae are resting against the intercondylar sulci, obscuring the patellofemoral joint spaces.

_____

313. The tibial tuberosities are demonstrated within the patellofemoral joint spaces. The patient's calves were not large.

_____

For the following tangential (axial) knee projections with poor positioning, state which anatomic structures are misaligned and how the patient should be repositioned for an optimal projection to be obtained.

Figure 6-82

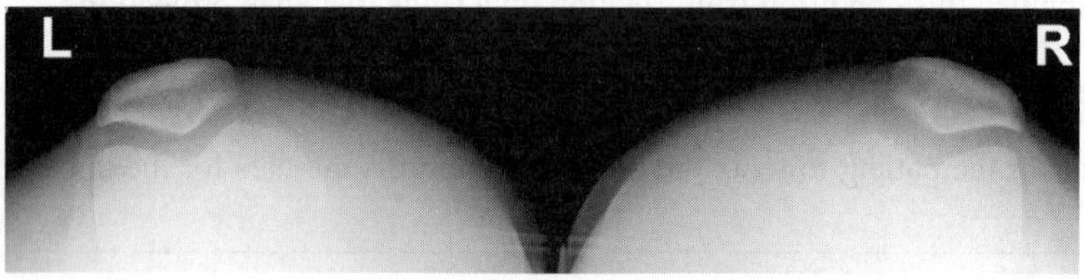

314. Figure 6-82: _____

_____

_____

_____

Figure 6-83

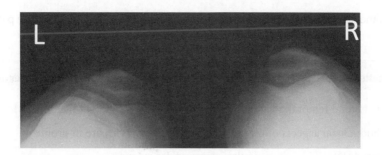

315. Figure 6-83: _____
_____
_____
_____

Figure 6-84

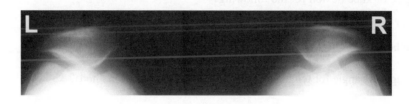
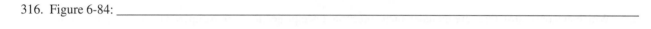

316. Figure 6-84: _____
_____
_____
_____

Figure 6-85

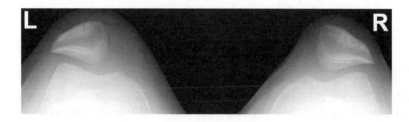

317. Figure 6-85: _____
_____
_____
_____

318. Complete the statements below referring to tangential (Inferosuperior; Settegast method) patella projection analysis guidelines.

Patella and Patellofemoral Joint: Tangential Projection (Inferosuperior and Settegast Method)
■ Inferosuperior: Lateral femoral condyle demonstrates (A) _____ height than the (B) _____ condyle.
■ Settegast method: Distal aspects of the (C) _____ condyles are in profile.
■ Patella is centered (D) _____ to the intercondylar sulcus.
■ The (E) _____ is at the center of the exposure field.
■ The (F) _____ and (G) _____ are seen with minimal distortion.

319. What is the degree of knee flexion for the following?

   A. Inferosuperior projection: _____

   B. Settegast method: _____

320. What is the average CR angle for tangential knee projection (Settegast method)?

   _____

321. Which anatomic structures are included on a tangential knee projection (inferosuperior) with accurate positioning?

   _____

   _____

For the following descriptions of tangential knee projections with poor positioning, state how the patient would have been mispositioned for such a projection to be obtained.

322. A portion of the proximal lower leg does not superimpose the distal femur, and the patella is lateral to the intercondylar sulcus.

   _____

323. Settegast method: the femoral condyles are at the same height, the patellofemoral joint space is closed, and the anterior tibia is at a distance greater than 0.125 inch (0.3 cm) distal from the intercondylar sulcus.

   _____

324. Inferosuperior: the lateral femoral condyle demonstrates more height than the medial condyle, the patellofemoral joint space is closed, and the anterior tibia is at a distance greater than 0.125 inch (0.3 cm) distal from the intercondylar sulcus.

   _____

For the following tangential (inferosuperior and Settegast Method) knee projections with poor positioning, state which anatomic structures are misaligned and how the patient should be repositioned for an optimal projection to be obtained.

Figure 6-86

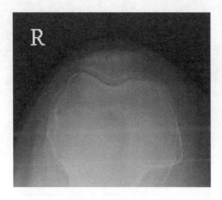

325. Figure 6-86, inferosuperior: _____

_____

_____

Figure 6-87

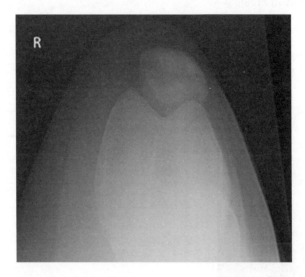

326. Figure 6-87, Settegast: _____

_____

_____

Figure 6-88

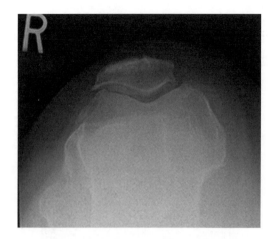

327. Figure 6-88, Settegast: _____

_____

_____

Femur: AP Projection

328. Identify the labeled anatomy in Figure 6-89.

Figure 6-89

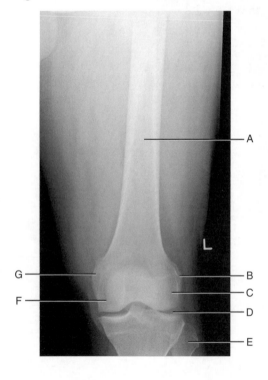

A. _____

B. _____

C. _____

D. _____

E. _____

F. _____

G. _____

329. Identify the labeled anatomy in Figure 6-90.

Figure 6-90

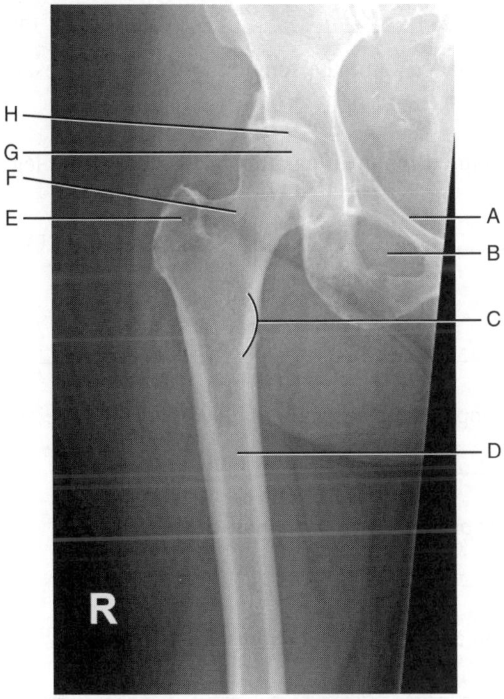

A. _____

B. _____

C. _____

D. _____

E. _____

F. _____

G. _____

H. _____

330. Complete the statements below referring to AP distal femur projection analysis guidelines.

AP Distal Femur Projection Analysis Guidelines
■ The medial and lateral epicondyles are in (A) _____, the femoral condyles are symmetrical in shape, and the tibia superimposes one-half of the (B) _____.   ■ The (C) _____ is at the center of the exposure field.

331. Complete the statements below referring to AP proximal femur projection analysis guidelines.

AP Proximal Femur Projection Analysis Guidelines
■ The ischial spine is aligned with the (A) _____, and the obturator foramen is open.   ■ The femoral neck is demonstrated without foreshortening, the (B) _____ trochanter is in profile laterally, and the (C) _____ trochanter is completely superimposed by the proximal femur.   ■ The (D) _____ is at the center of the exposure field.

332. How is the femur positioned with respect to the x-ray tube for an AP femoral projection to take advantage of the anode-heel effect?

_____

333. Why is it necessary to include all the femoral soft tissue when imaging the femur?

_____

334. An AP distal femur is obtained by placing the patient in a(n) (A) _____ position with the knee (B) _____ and leg (C) _____ rotated until the femoral epicondyles are at equal distances from the IR.

335. Should the technologist rotate a patient with a suspected fractured femur in an attempt to position the leg in an AP projection?

A. _____ (Yes/No)

Justify your answer.

B. _____

336. Accurate CR centering on a distal femoral projection is accomplished by positioning the lower IR edge approximately (A) _____ inch(es) below the (B) _____ joint.

337. Which anatomic structures are included on an AP distal femur projection with accurate positioning?

_____

338. How can the patient be positioned to prevent pelvic rotation on an AP proximal femur projection?

_____

339. How are the femoral epicondyles positioned for an AP proximal femur projection?

A. _____

How will this positioning demonstrate the femoral neck and greater trochanter on the resulting projection?

B. _____

340. On an AP proximal femur projection with accurate positioning, the (A) _____ is centered within the exposure field. This is accomplished by placing the upper IR edge at the level of the (B) _____.

341. Which anatomic structures are included on an AP proximal femur projection with accurate positioning?

_____

For the following descriptions of AP femoral projections with poor positioning, state how the patient would have been mispositioned for such a projection to be obtained.

342. Distal femur: The medial femoral condyle appears larger than the lateral condyle, and the intercondylar eminence is not centered within the intercondylar fossa.

_____

343. Proximal femur: The affected side's obturator foramen is narrowed, and the iliac spine is demonstrated without pelvic brim superimposition.

_____

344. Proximal femur: The affected side's obturator foramen is open, and the ischial spine is not aligned with the pelvic brim but is demonstrated closer to the acetabulum.

_____

345. Proximal femur: The femoral neck is partially foreshortened, and the lesser trochanter is demonstrated in profile.

_____

For the following AP femoral projections with poor positioning, state which anatomic structures are misaligned and how the patient should be repositioned for an optimal projection to be obtained.

Figure 6-91

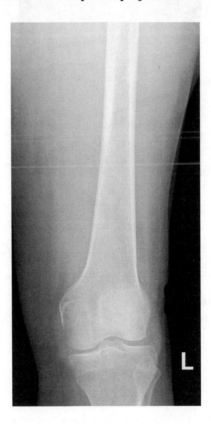

346. Figure 6-91, distal femur: _____

_____

_____

_____

Figure 6-92

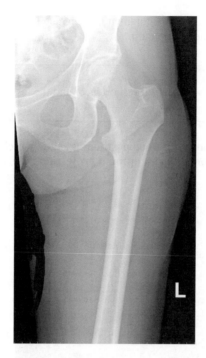

347. Figure 6-92, proximal femur: _____

_____

_____

_____

Femur: Lateral Projection (Mediolateral)

348. Identify the labeled anatomy in Figure 6-93.

Figure 6-93

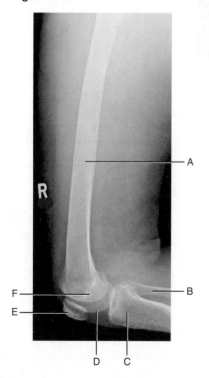

A. _____

B. _____

C. _____

D. _____

E. _____

F. _____

349. Identify the labeled anatomy in Figure 6-94.

Figure 6-94

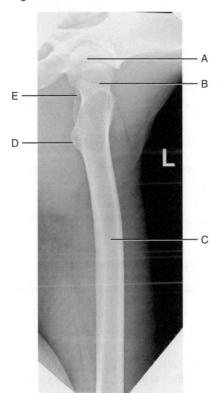

A. _____

B. _____

C. _____

D. _____

E. _____

350. Identify the labeled anatomy in Figure 6-95.

Figure 6-95

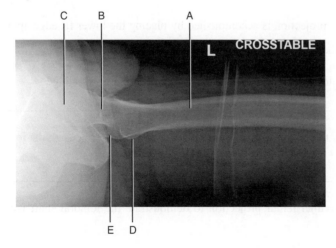

A. _____

B. _____

C. _____

D. _____

E. _____

Chapter **6 Image Analysis of the Lower Extremity**

351. Complete the statements below referring to lateral distal femur projection analysis guidelines.

Lateral Distal Femur Projection Analysis Guidelines
■ Anterior and posterior margins of the (A) _____ and (B) _____ condyles are aligned.
■ The (C) _____ is at the center of the exposure field.

352. Complete the statements below referring to lateral proximal femur projection analysis guidelines.

Lateral Proximal Femur Projection Analysis Guidelines
■ The lesser trochanter is in profile (A) _____, and the femoral neck and head are superimposed over the (B) _____.
■ The femoral shaft is seen without foreshortening, the femoral neck is demonstrated on end, and the (C) _____ trochanter is demonstrated at the same transverse level as the femoral head.
■ The (D) _____ is at the center of the exposure field.

353. A lateral distal femur projection is obtained by rotating the patient onto the (A) _____ (medial/lateral) aspect of the affected femur until an imaginary line connecting the femoral epicondyles is aligned (B) _____ to the IR.

354. How is a lateral distal femur projection obtained in a patient with a known or suspected femur fracture?

_____

355. Accurate CR centering on a lateral distal femur projection is accomplished by placing the lower IR edge approximately (A) _____ inch(es) below the (B) _____.

356. Which anatomic structures are included on a lateral distal femur projection with accurate positioning?

_____

357. How is the patient positioned to place the lesser trochanter in profile and the greater trochanter beneath the femoral neck on a lateral proximal femur projection?

_____

358. How is the patient positioned for a lateral proximal femur projection to demonstrate the femoral shaft without foreshortening and the femoral neck on end?

_____

359. What position is performed to demonstrate a lateral proximal femur when a fracture is suspected or known to be present?

_____

360. On a lateral proximal femoral projection with accurate positioning, the (A) _____ is centered within the collimated field. This is accomplished by positioning the upper IR edge at the level of the (B) _____.

361. Which anatomic structures are included on a lateral proximal femoral projection with accurate positioning?

_____

For the following descriptions of lateral femoral projections with poor positioning, state how the patient would have been mispositioned for such a projection to be obtained.

362. Distal femur: The anterior and posterior surfaces of the medial and lateral femoral condyles are demonstrated without alignment. The medial condyle is posterior to the lateral condyle.

_____

363. Proximal femur: The greater trochanter is demonstrated medially (next to the ischial tuberosity), and the lesser trochanter is obscured.

_____

364. Proximal femur: The greater trochanter is demonstrated laterally, and the lesser trochanter is obscured.

_____

For the following lateral femoral projections with poor positioning, state which anatomic structures are misaligned and how the patient should be repositioned for an optimal projection to be obtained.

Figure 6-96

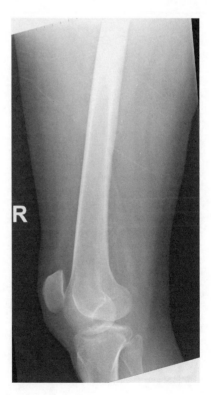

365. Figure 6-96, distal femur: _____

_____

_____

_____

Figure 6-97

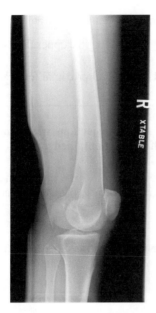

366. Figure 6-97, trauma lateromedial distal femur: _____

_____

_____

_____

Figure 6-98

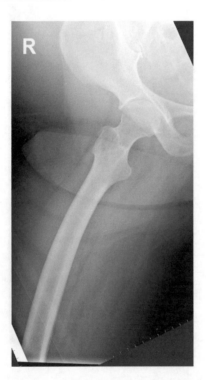

367. Figure 6-98, proximal femur: _____

_____

_____

_____

Figure 6-99

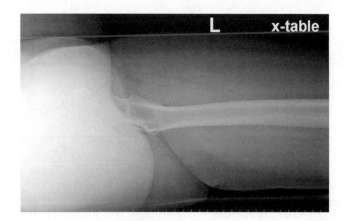

368. Figure 6-99, proximal femur: _____

_____

_____

_____

Figure 6-100

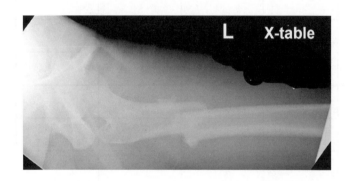

369. Figure 6-100, trauma proximal femur: _____

_____

_____

_____

7 Image Analysis of the Hip and Pelvis

STUDY QUESTIONS

1. Complete Figure 7-1.

   Figure 7-1

Projection	kV	Grid	AEC	mAs	SID
AP, pelvis					
AP frog-leg, pelvis					
AP oblique pelvis (Judet method)					
AP axial outlet pelvis (Taylor method)					
Superoinferior axial inlet pelvis					
AP, hip					
AP frog-leg, hip					
Axiolateral (inferosuperior), hip					
AP axial, sacroiliac joints					
AP oblique, sacroiliac joints					
Pediatric					

2. List the four soft tissue structures that are demonstrated on accurately exposed AP hip and pelvis projections and describe their locations.

   A. _____

   B. _____

   C. _____

   D. _____

   Why is it important that these soft tissue structures are visualized?

   E. _____

Pelvis: AP Projection

3. Identify the labeled anatomy in Figure 7-2.

Figure 7-2

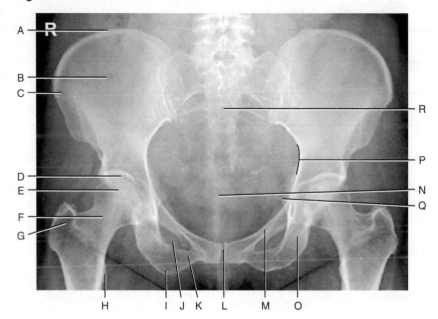

A. _____	J. _____
B. _____	K. _____
C. _____	L. _____
D. _____	M. _____
E. _____	N. _____
F. _____	O. _____
G. _____	P. _____
H. _____	Q. _____
I. _____	R. _____

4. Complete Figure 7-3.

Figure 7-3

Male and Female Pelvic Differences		
Parameter	Male	Female
Overall shape		
Ala (iliac wing)		
Pubic arch angle		
Inlet shape		
Obturator foramen		

5. Complete the statements below referring to AP pelvis projection analysis guidelines.

AP Pelvis Projection Analysis Guidelines

■ The (A) _____ and coccyx are aligned with the pubis symphysis, and the obturator foramina are open and uniform in size and shape.

■ The femoral necks are demonstrated without foreshortening, the (B) _____ trochanters are in profile laterally, and the (C) _____ trochanters are superimposed by the femoral necks.

---

6. State whether the following pelvis projections are from a female or male patient:

Figure 7-4

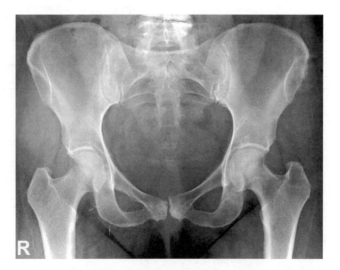

A. Figure 7-4: _____

Figure 7-5

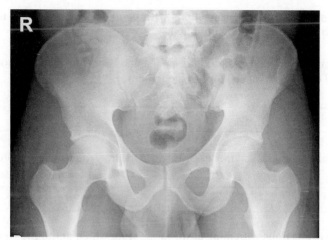

B. Figure 7-5: _____

7. How can patient positioning be evaluated to ensure that pelvic rotation is not present on an AP pelvic projection?

_____

8. Describe the relationship of the sacrum and coccyx to the pubis symphysis and the symmetry of the iliac wings and obturator foramen on an AP pelvic projection in which the patient's left side was rotated away (RPO) from the IR.

_____

_____

9. Following are descriptions of the femoral neck appearance on different AP pelvic projections. For each description, state the position of the patient's feet and femoral epicondyles that would result in the described projection.

A. Femoral necks without foreshortening: _____

_____

B. Femoral necks on end: _____

_____

C. Femoral necks partially foreshortened: _____

_____

10. How are the patient's feet and femoral epicondyles positioned for an AP pelvic projection with accurate positioning to be obtained?

_____

_____

11. Accurate CR centering on an AP pelvic projection is accomplished by centering a(n) (A) _____ CR to the midsagittal plane at a level halfway between the (B) _____ and an imaginary line connecting the (C) _____.

12. Which anatomic structures are included on an AP pelvic projection with accurate positioning?

_____

For the following descriptions of AP pelvic projections with poor positioning, state how the patient would have been mispositioned for such a projection to be obtained.

13. The right obturator foramen is narrowed, the right ischial spine is demonstrated without pelvic brim superimposition, and the sacrum and coccyx are rotated toward the left hip.

_____

_____

14. The femoral necks are foreshortened, and the lesser trochanters are demonstrated in profile.

_____

_____

For the following AP pelvic projections with poor positioning, state which anatomic structures are misaligned and how the patient should be repositioned for an optimal projection to be obtained.

Figure 7-6

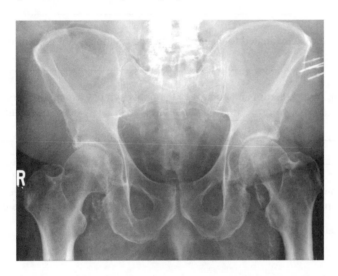

15. Figure 7-6: _____

_____

_____

_____

_____

Figure 7-7

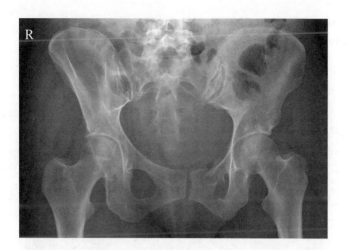

16. Figure 7-7: _____

_____

_____

_____

Figure 7-8

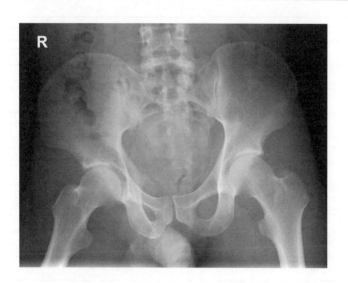

17. Figure 7-8: _____

_____

_____

_____

Pelvis: AP Frogleg Projection (Modified Cleaves Method)

18. Identify the labeled anatomy in Figure 7-9.

Figure 7-9

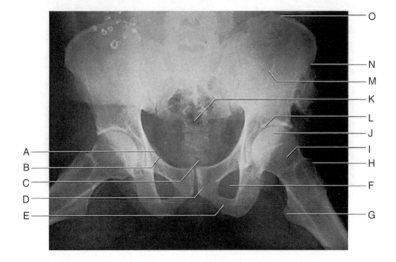

A. _____

B. _____

C. _____

D. _____

E. _____

F. _____

G. _____

H. _____

I. _____

J. _____

K. _____

L. _____

M. _____

N. _____

O. _____

19. Complete the statements below referring to AP frogleg pelvis projection analysis guidelines.

AP Frogleg (Modified Cleaves Method) Pelvis Projection Analysis Guidelines
■ The sacrum and coccyx are aligned with the pubis symphysis, the (A) _____ are symmetrical, and the obturator foramina are partially foreshortened and uniform in size and shape.
■ The lesser trochanters are in profile (B) _____, and the (C) _____ are superimposed over the adjacent greater trochanters.
■ The femoral necks are partially foreshortened, and the (D) _____ are demonstrated at the same transverse level halfway between the femoral heads and lesser trochanters.

Chapter **7 Image Analysis of the Hip and Pelvis**

20. The degree of patient knee and hip flexion determines the position of the greater and lesser trochanters to the

_____.

21. At what degree with the imaging table are the femurs placed to accurately position the greater and lesser trochanters on an AP frogleg pelvic projection?

_____

22. The patient's knees and hips were flexed 20 degrees with the imaging table for an AP frogleg pelvic projection. How can this positioning error be identified on the resulting projection?

_____

23. The degree of femoral abduction for an AP frogleg pelvic projection determines which two anatomic relationships?

A. _____

B. _____

24. Describe the position of the greater trochanters and the degree of femoral neck foreshortening that are demonstrated on an AP frogleg pelvic projection if the femurs are abducted as follows:

A. Femurs are abducted until placed against the imaging table:

_____

B. Femurs are abducted to a 45-degree angle with the imaging table:

_____

C. Femurs are abducted only 20 to 30 degrees from vertical:

_____

25. Accurate CR centering on an AP frogleg pelvic projection is accomplished by centering a(n) (A) _____

CR to the (B) _____ plane at a level (C) _____ superior to the (D) _____.

26. Which anatomic structures are included on an AP frogleg pelvic projection with accurate positioning?

_____

For the following descriptions of AP frogleg pelvic projections with poor positioning, state how the patient would have been mispositioned for such a projection to be obtained.

27. The left obturator foramen is narrowed, the left iliac wing is wider than the right, and the sacrum and coccyx are rotated toward the right hip.

_____

28. The femoral necks are demonstrated on end, and the greater trochanters are demonstrated on the same transverse level as the femoral heads.

_____

For the following AP frogleg pelvic projections with poor positioning, state which anatomic structures are misaligned and how the patient should be repositioned for an optimal projection to be obtained.

Figure 7-10

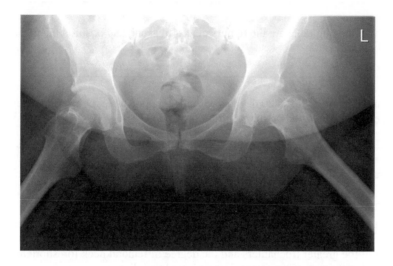

29. Figure 7-10: _____

_____

_____

_____

Figure 7-11

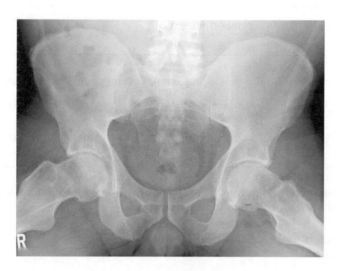

30. Figure 7-11: _____

_____

_____

_____

Figure 7-12

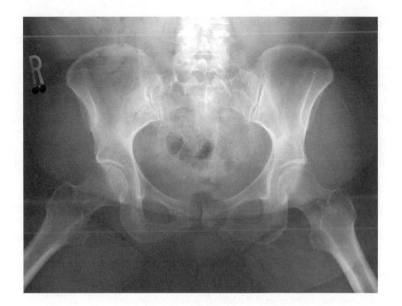

31. Figure 7-12: _____

_____

_____

_____

Figure 7-13

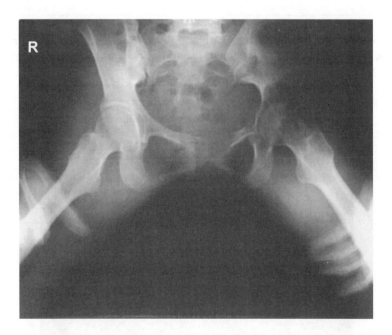

32. Figure 7-13: _____

_____

_____

_____

Pelvis (Acetabulum) AP Oblique Projection (Judet Method)

33. Complete the statements below referring to AP oblique pelvis projection analysis guidelines.

AP Oblique Pelvis Projection Analysis Guidelines

- The side-up hip demonstrates the (A) _____ on end and the

  (B) _____body superimposed.

- Side-down hip demonstrates the iliac wing without (C) _____, and the ilioischial column and

  (D) _____ rim of the acetabulum are demonstrated.

---

34. Which body plane is used to determine patient obliquity for an AP oblique pelvis projection?

    A. _____

    How much is the patient torso rotated for an AP oblique pelvis projection?

    B. _____

35. Accurate CR centering on an AP oblique pelvis projection is accomplished by centering the CR 2 inches (5 cm)

    (A) _____ to elevated ASIS, at the level of the (B) _____.

36. Which anatomic structures are included on an AP oblique pelvis projection with accurate positioning?

    _____

For the following AP oblique pelvis projection with poor positioning, state which anatomic structures are misaligned and how the patient should be repositioned for an optimal projection to be obtained.

Figure 7-14

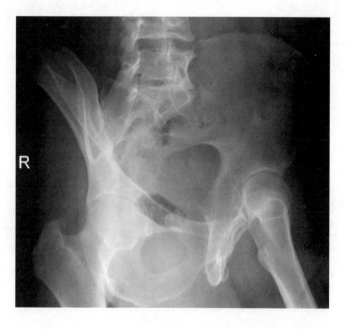

37. Figure 7-14: _____

    _____

Pelvis (Anterior Pelvic Bones): AP Axial Outlet Projection (Taylor Method)

38. Complete the statements below referring to AP axial outlet pelvis projection analysis guidelines.

AP Axial Outlet Pelvis Projection Analysis Guidelines

- The sacrum and coccyx are aligned with the (A) _____, and the (B) _____are symmetrical.

- Pubic bone (C) _____ the 3-4 sacral segments, and the ischial spines are centered within the

  (D) _____.

39. How is the CR positioned to demonstrate the superior and inferior rami of the pelvis, ischial rami, and obturator foramina without longitudinal foreshortening?

   A. For a male patient: _____

   B. For a female patient: _____

40. Accurate CR centering on an AP axial outlet pelvis projection is obtained by positioning the CR to a midline point

   (A) _____inches (B) _____ to the superior border of the (C) _____.

For the following AP axial outlet pelvis projection with poor positioning, state which anatomic structures are misaligned and how the patient should be repositioned for an optimal projection to be obtained.

Figure 7-15

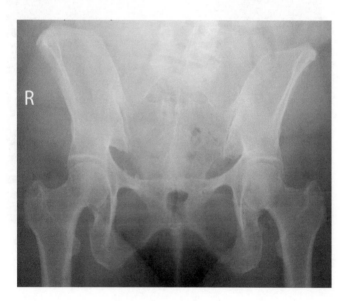

41. Figure 7-15:_____

_____

Pelvis (Anterior Pelvic Bones): Superoinferior Axial Inlet Projection (Bridgeman Method)

42. Complete the statements below referring to superoinferior axial inlet pelvis projection analysis guidelines.

Superoinferior Axial Inlet Pelvis Projection Analysis Guidelines
■ Ischial spines are symmetrically demonstrated within the (A) _____.
■ Superior and inferior pubic rami are (B) _____ closing the obturator foramina. The (C) _____ is demonstrated without foreshortening. Ischial spines are at the (D)_____ level as the coccyx.

43. How is the CR positioned to demonstrate the ischial spines at the same level as the coccyx? _____

_____

44. Accurate CR centering on a superoinferior axial inlet pelvis projection is obtained by positioning the CR to the

patient's (A) _____ plane at the level of the (B) _____.

For the following superoinferior axial inlet pelvis projection with poor positioning, state which anatomic structures are misaligned and how the patient should be repositioned for an optimal projection to be obtained.

Figure 7-16

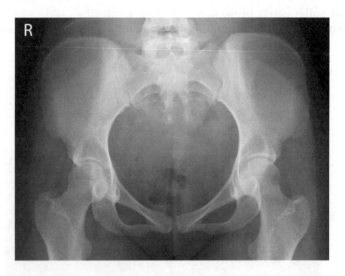

45. Figure 7-16:_____

_____

Hip: AP Projection

46. Identify the labeled anatomy in Figure 7-17.

Figure 7-17

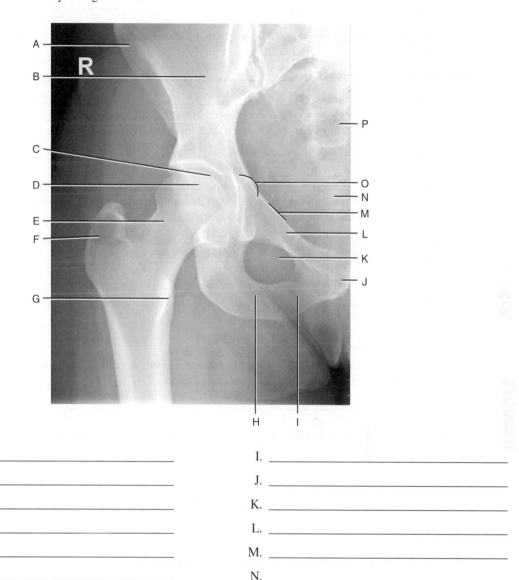

A. _____   I. _____

B. _____   J. _____

C. _____   K. _____

D. _____   L. _____

E. _____   M. _____

F. _____   N. _____

G. _____   O. _____

H. _____   P. _____

47. Complete the statements below referring to AP hip projection analysis guidelines.

AP Hip Projection Analysis Guidelines

■ The (A) _____ and coccyx are aligned with the (B) _____, and the obturator foramen is open.

■ The femoral neck is demonstrated without foreshortening, the greater trochanter is in profile (C) _____, and the lesser trochanter is superimposed by the (D) _____.

---

48. How can patient positioning be evaluated to ensure that pelvic rotation is not present on an AP hip projection?

_____

49. Describe the relationship that would result between the following anatomic structures on an AP hip projection if the affected side was rotated away from the IR.

A. Sacrum and symphysis pubis: _____

B. Ischial spine and pelvic brim: _____

50. If the affected hip is rotated toward the IR for an AP hip projection, how will the obturator foramen appear in

comparison with a nonrotated AP hip projection? _____

51. The demonstration of the femoral neck and lesser trochanter on an AP hip projection depends on the position of the femoral epicondyles. For each epicondyle position in the following list, describe how the femoral neck and lesser trochanter are demonstrated on an AP hip projection:

A. The leg is externally rotated, with the foot at a 45-degree angle and an imaginary line connecting the femoral epicondyles at a 60- to 65-degree angle with the imaging table:

_____

B. The leg is internally rotated, with the foot vertical and an imaginary line connecting the femoral epicondyles at a 15- to 20-degree angle with the imaging table:

_____

C. The leg is internally rotated, with the foot 15 to 20 degrees from vertical and an imaginary line connecting the femoral epicondyles aligned parallel with the imaging table:

_____

52. How are the patient's foot and femoral epicondyles positioned to obtain an AP hip projection with accurate positioning?

_____

53. Should the technologist attempt to rotate the leg of a patient with a suspected fracture or dislocated hip?

A. _____ (Yes/No)

54. To center the femoral head in the center of the exposure field, a(n) (A) _____ CR is centered 1.5 inches

(4 cm) (B) _____ to the midpoint of a line connecting the ASIS and (C) _____.

55. Which anatomic structures are included on an AP hip projection with accurate positioning?

_____

56. How may the positioning procedure require adjusting if the patient has a prosthesis?

_____

For the following descriptions of AP hip projections with poor positioning, state how the patient would have been mispositioned for such a projection to be obtained.

57. The ischial spine is demonstrated without pelvic brim superimposition, the sacrum and coccyx are not aligned with the symphysis pubis but are rotated away from the affected hip, and the obturator foramen is narrowed.

_____

_____

58. The ischial spine is not aligned with the pelvic brim but is demonstrated closer to the acetabulum, the sacrum and coccyx are not aligned with the symphysis pubis but are rotated toward the affected hip, and the obturator foramen is clearly demonstrated.

_____

_____

59. The femoral neck is completely foreshortened, and the lesser trochanter is demonstrated in profile.

_____

_____

For the following AP hip projections with poor positioning, state which anatomic structures are misaligned and how the patient should be repositioned for an optimal projection to be obtained.

Figure 7-18

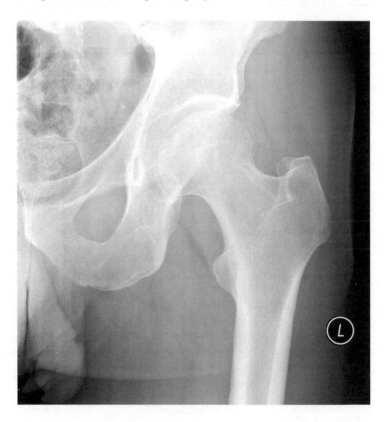

60. Figure 7-18: _____

_____

_____

_____

Chapter **7 Image Analysis of the Hip and Pelvis**

Figure 7-19

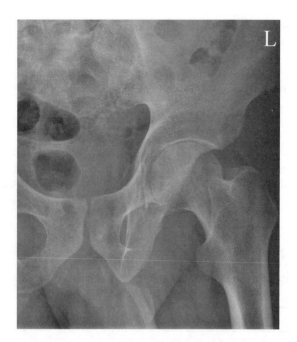

61. Figure 7-19: _____

_____

_____

_____

Figure 7-20

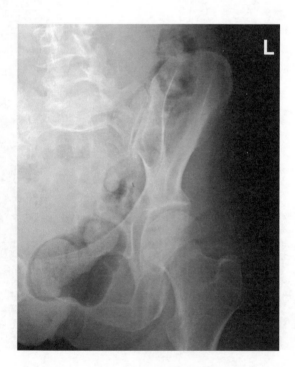

62. Figure 7-20: _____

_____

_____

_____

Chapter **7 Image Analysis of the Hip and Pelvis**

Figure 7-21

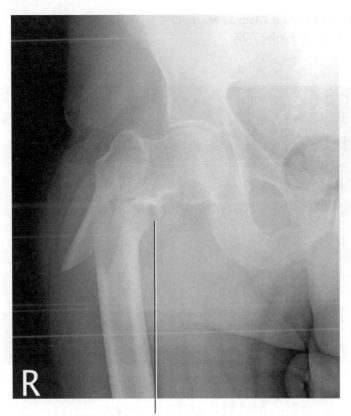

Lesser trochanter

63. Figure 7-21, fracture: _____

_____

_____

_____

_____

Hip: AP Frogleg Projection (Modified Cleaves Method)

64. Identify the labeled anatomy in Figure 7-22.

Figure 7-22

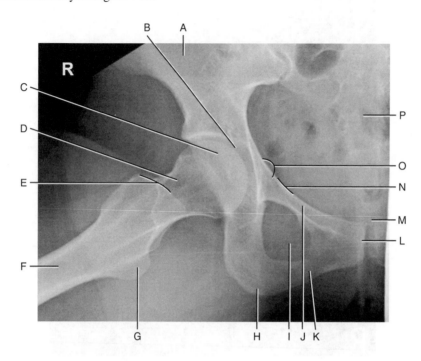

A. _____

B. _____

C. _____

D. _____

E. _____

F. _____

G. _____

H. _____

I. _____

J. _____

K. _____

L. _____

M. _____

N. _____

O. _____

P. _____

65. For the Lauenstein and Hickey lateral hip methods, the patient's pelvis is rotated (A) _____ (toward/ away from) the affected hip until the femur is placed (B) _____.

66. The degree of patient knee and hip flexion determines whether or not the greater and lesser trochanter will be in

_____.

67. At what degree with the imaging table is the femur placed to accurately position the greater and lesser trochanters on an AP frogleg hip projection? _____

68. The degree of femoral abduction for an AP frogleg hip projection will determine which two proximal femur anatomic relationships?

A. _____

B. _____

348

69. Describe the position of the greater trochanter and the degree of femoral neck foreshortening demonstrated on an AP frogleg hip projection if the femur is abducted as stated for each of the following:

A. The femur is abducted until it is placed next to the imaging table:

_____

B. The femur is abducted to a 45-degree angle with the imaging table:

_____

C. The femur is abducted 20 to 30 degrees from vertical:

_____

70. Accurate CR centering on an AP frogleg hip projection is accomplished by centering a(n) (A) _____ CR (B) _____ inch(es) distal to the midpoint of a line connecting the (C) _____ and pubis symphysis.

71. Which anatomic structures are included on an AP frogleg hip projection with accurate positioning?

_____

For the following descriptions of AP frogleg hip projections with poor positioning, state how the patient would have been mispositioned for such a projection to be obtained.

72. The ischial spine is demonstrated without pelvic brim superimposition, the sacrum and coccyx are not aligned with the symphysis pubis but are rotated away from the affected hip, and the obturator foramen is narrowed.

_____

73. The greater trochanter is positioned medially, and the lesser trochanter is obscured.

_____

74. The greater trochanter is positioned laterally.

_____

75. The femoral neck is demonstrated on end, and the greater trochanter is demonstrated on the same transverse level as the femoral head.

_____

For the following AP frogleg hip projections with poor positioning, state which anatomic structures are misaligned and how the patient should be repositioned for an optimal projection to be obtained.

Figure 7-23

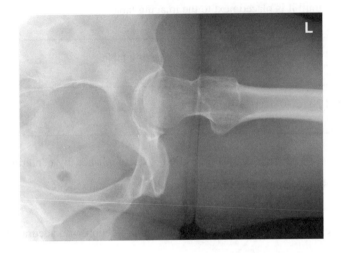

76. Figure 7-23: _____

_____

_____

_____

Figure 7-24

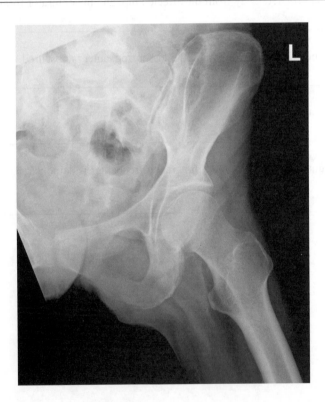

77. Figure 7-24: _____

_____

_____

_____

Figure 7-25

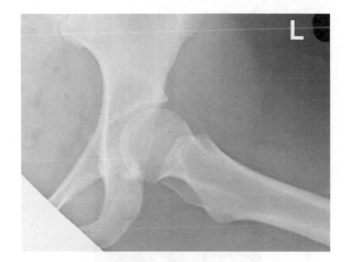

78. Figure 7-25: _____

_____

_____

_____

Figure 7-26

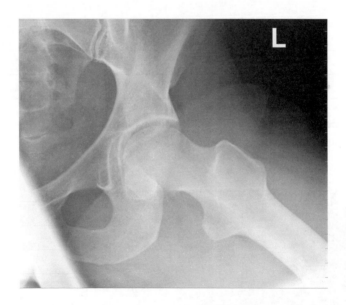

79. Figure 7-26: _____

_____

_____

_____

Figure 7-27

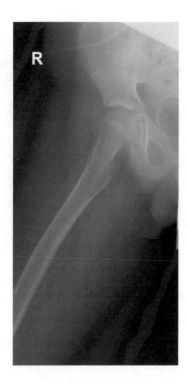

80. Figure 7-27: _____

_____

_____

_____

Hip: Axiolateral (Inferosuperior) Projection (Danelius-Miller Method)

81. Identify the labeled anatomy in Figure 7-28.

Figure 7-28

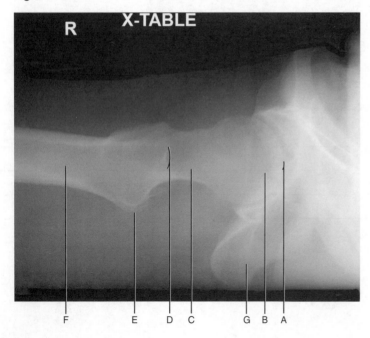

A. _____

B. _____

C. _____

D. _____

E. _____

F. _____

G. _____

82. Complete the statements below referring to the AP frogleg hip projection analysis guidelines.

AP Frogleg (Modified Cleaves Method) Hip Projection Analysis Guidelines
■ The (A) _____ is aligned with the pelvic brim, the sacrum and coccyx are aligned with the pubis symphysis, and the obturator foramina is partially foreshortened.
■ The (B) _____ is in profile medially, and the (C) _____ is superimposed over the greater trochanter.
■ The (D) _____ is partially foreshortened, and the proximal (E) _____ is demonstrated at a transverse level halfway between the femoral head and the lesser trochanter.

83. Complete the statements below referring to axiolateral hip projection analysis guidelines.

Axiolateral Hip Projection Analysis Guidelines
■ The femoral neck is demonstrated without foreshortening, and the (A) _____ are demonstrated at approximately the same level.
■ The lesser trochanter is in profile (B) _____, and the greater trochanter is superimposed by the (C) _____.

84. State three ways that the amount of scatter radiation reaching the IR can be reduced on an axiolateral hip projection.

A. _____

B. _____

C. _____

85. How is the unaffected leg positioned for an axiolateral hip projection to prevent its soft tissue from superimposing the affected hip?

_____

86. Where is the grid-IR placed for an axiolateral hip projection?

A. _____

How is it aligned with the femoral neck?

B. _____

How is the position of the grid-IR changed if the patient has a large amount of lateral soft tissue thickness?

C. _____

How should the CR be positioned with respect to the IR and femoral neck?

D. _____

87. Describe how to localize the femoral neck when positioning for an axiolateral hip projection.

_____

Chapter **7 Image Analysis of the Hip and Pelvis**

88. Describe the appearance of the femoral neck and greater trochanter if the CR is too large to accurately align it with the femoral neck for an axiolateral hip projection.

A. Femoral neck: _____

B. Greater trochanter: _____

89. How is the leg positioned to accurately place the lesser trochanter on an axiolateral hip projection?

_____

90. On an axiolateral hip projection with accurate positioning, the _____ is centered within the collimated field.

91. Which anatomic structures are included on an axiolateral hip projection with accurate positioning?

_____

For the following descriptions of axiolateral hip projections with poor positioning, state how the patient or CR would have been mispositioned for such a projection to be obtained.

92. The soft tissue from the unaffected thigh is superimposed over the acetabulum and femoral head of the affected hip.

_____

93. The greater trochanter is demonstrated at a transverse level that is proximal to the lesser trochanter, and the femoral neck is partially foreshortened.

_____

94. The greater trochanter is demonstrated posteriorly, and the lesser trochanter is superimposed over the femoral shaft.

_____

For the following axiolateral hip projections with poor positioning, state which anatomic structures are misaligned and how the patient or CR should be repositioned for an optimal projection to be obtained.

Figure 7-29

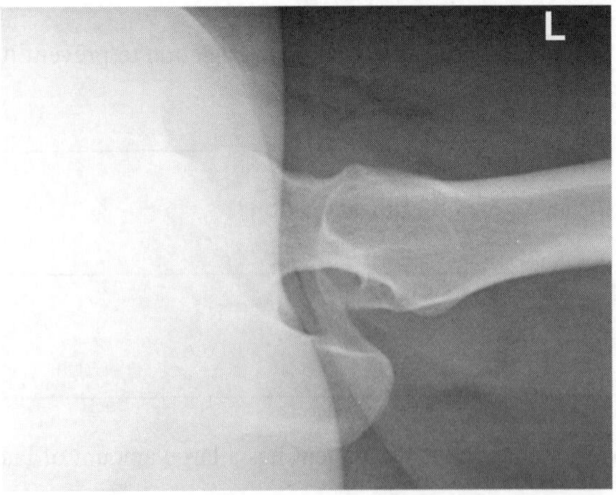

95. Figure 7-29: _____

_____

_____

_____

_____

Figure 7-30

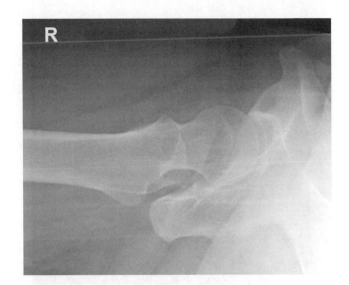

96. Figure 7-30: _____

_____

_____

_____

Figure 7-31

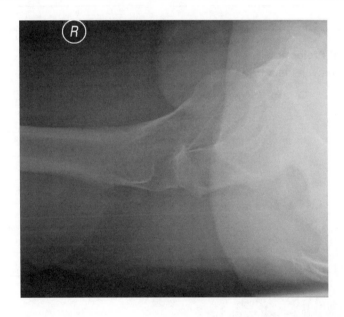

97. Figure 7-31: _____

_____

_____

_____

Figure 7-32

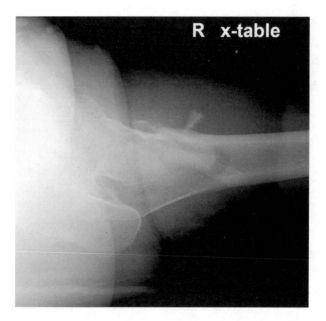

98. Figure 7-32, fracture: _____

_____

_____

_____

Sacroiliac Joints: AP Axial Projection

99. Identify the labeled anatomy in Figure 7-33.

Figure 7-33

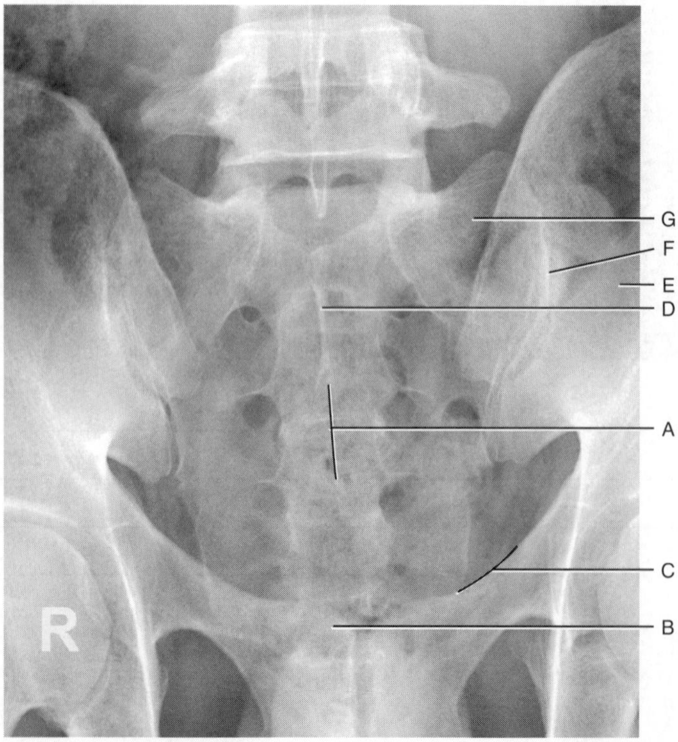

A. _____

B. _____

C. _____

D. _____

E. _____

F. _____

G. _____

100. Complete the statements below referring to AP axial sacroiliac joints projection analysis guidelines.

AP Axial Sacroiliac Joints Projection Analysis Guidelines

- The median sacral crest is aligned with the (A) _____, and the sacrum is at equal distance from the lateral wall of the pelvic brim on both sides.
- The sacroiliac joints are demonstrated without foreshortening, and the sacrum is elongated, with the (B) _____ superimposed over the fifth sacral segments.

---

101. When a patient is rotated for an AP axial sacroiliac joint projection, the sacrum rotates in the (A) _____ (same/opposite) direction as the pubis symphysis and is positioned next to the lateral wall of the pelvic brim situated (B) _____ (closer to/farther from) the IR.

102. How are the patient and CR positioned to demonstrate the sacroiliac joints without foreshortening?

A. For a male patient: _____

B. For a female patient: _____

C. For a patient with greater than average lumbosacral curvature: _____

D. For a patient with less than average lumbosacral curvature: _____

103. Why is the median sacral crest aligned with the long axis of the collimated field for an AP axial sacroiliac joint projection?

_____

104. Accurate CR centering on an AP axial sacroiliac joint projection is obtained by positioning the CR to the patient's (A) _____ plane at a level (B) _____ superior to the pubis symphysis.

105. Which anatomic structures are included on an AP axial sacroiliac joint projection with accurate positioning?

_____

For the following descriptions of sacroiliac joint projections with poor positioning, state how the patient or CR would have been mispositioned for such a projection to be obtained.

106. The sacrum is situated closer to the right pelvic brim than to the left.

_____

107. The sacroiliac joints are foreshortened, and the inferior sacrum is demonstrated without pubis symphysis superimposition.

_____

For the following AP axial sacroiliac joint projections with poor positioning, state which anatomic structures are misaligned and how the patient should be repositioned for an optimal projection to be obtained.

Figure 7-34

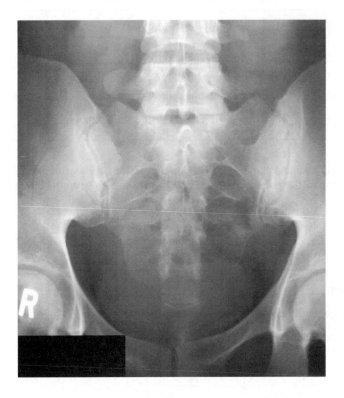

108. Figure 7-34: _____

_____

_____

_____

Figure 7-35

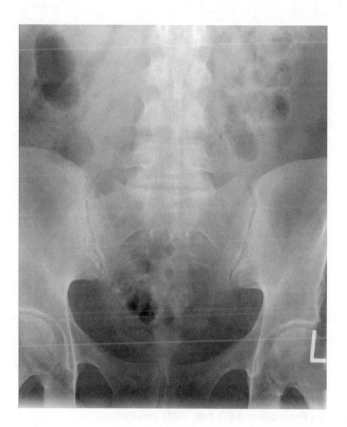

109. Figure 7-35: _____

_____

_____

_____

Figure 7-36

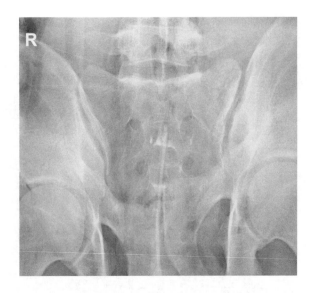

110. Figure 7-36: _____

_____

_____

_____

Sacroiliac Joints: AP Oblique Projection (LPO and RPO Positions)

111. Identify the labeled anatomy in Figure 7-37.

Figure 7-37

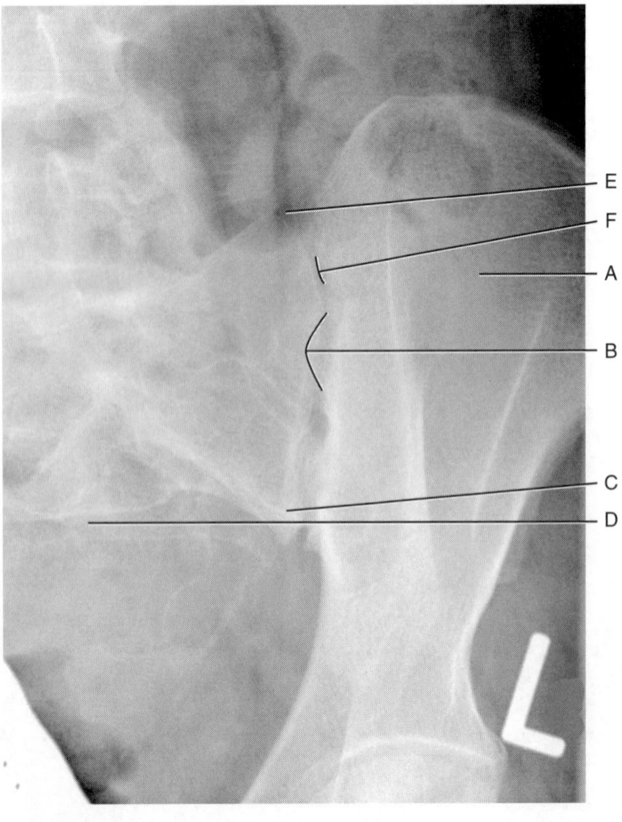

A. _____

B. _____

C. _____

D. _____

E. _____

F. _____

112. Complete the statements below referring to AP oblique sacroiliac joint projection analysis guidelines.

AP Oblique Sacroiliac Joints Projection Analysis Guidelines
■ The ilium and (A) _____ are demonstrated without superimposition, and the sacroiliac joint is open.
■ The long axis of the sacroiliac joint is aligned with the (B) _____ of the collimated field.

113. Which two bony structures articulate to form the sacroiliac joints?

    A. _____

    B. _____

114. For an open sacroiliac joint to be obtained on an AP oblique sacroiliac joint projection, the patient is rotated until

    the (A) _____ plane is at a (B) _____-degree angle with the IR.

115. Which sacroiliac joint is open when the patient is placed in an LPO position?

    _____

116. The affected sacroiliac joint is centered within the collimated field on an AP oblique sacroiliac joint projection with accurate positioning. This centering is obtained by placing the CR 1 inch (2.5 cm) (A) _____ (medial/

    lateral) to the elevated (B) _____.

117. Which anatomic structures are included on an AP oblique sacroiliac joint projection with accurate positioning?

    _____

    _____

For the following descriptions of AP oblique sacroiliac joint projections with poor positioning, state how the patient would have been mispositioned for such a projection to be obtained.

118. The sacroiliac joint is closed, the superior and inferior sacral ala are demonstrated without iliac superimposition, and the lateral sacral ala is superimposed over the iliac tuberosity.

    _____

119. The sacroiliac joint is closed, and the ilium is superimposed over the lateral sacral ala and inferior sacrum.

    _____

For the following sacroiliac joint projections with poor positioning, state which anatomic structures are misaligned and how the patient should be repositioned for an optimal projection to be obtained.

Figure 7-38

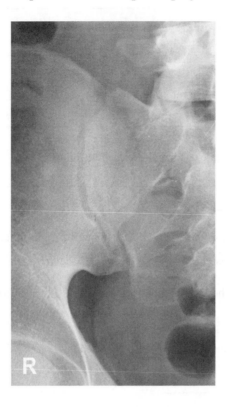

120. Figure 7-38: _____

_____

_____

_____

_____

Figure 7-39

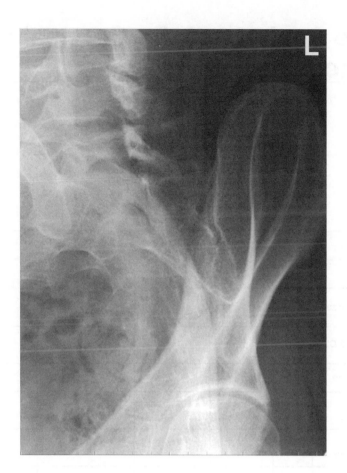

121. Figure 7-39: _____

_____

_____

_____

8 Image Analysis of the Cervical and Thoracic Vertebrae

STUDY QUESTIONS

1. Complete Figure 8-1.

Figure 8-1

Cervical and Thoracic Vertebrae Technical Data					
Projection	kV	Grid	AEC	mAs	**SID**
AP axial, cervical vertebrae					
AP, open-mouth, C1 and C2					
Lateral, cervical vertebrae					
PA or AP axial oblique, cervical vertebrae					
Lateral (Twining method), cervicothoracic vertebrae					
AP, thoracic vertebrae					
Lateral, thoracic vertebrae					
Pediatric					

Cervical Vertebrae: AP Axial Projection

2. Identify the labeled anatomy in Figure 8-2.

Figure 8-2

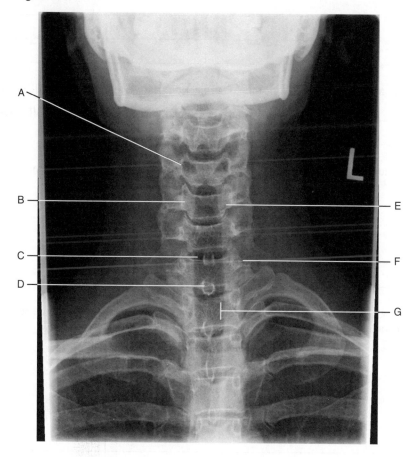

A. _____

B. _____

C. _____

D. _____

E. _____

F. _____

G. _____

3. Complete the statements below referring to AP axial cervical vertebrae projection analysis guidelines.

AP Axial Cervical Vertebrae Projection Analysis Guidelines

- The (A) _____ are aligned with the midline of the cervical bodies, the mandibular angles and mastoid tips are at equal distances from the cervical vertebrae, the articular pillars and pedicles are symmetrically visualized (B) _____ to the cervical bodies, and the distance from the vertebral column to the medial clavicular ends are equal.

- The intervertebral disk spaces are open, the vertebral bodies are demonstrated without distortion, and each vertebra's spinous process is visualized at the level of its (C) _____ intervertebral disk space.

- The third cervical vertebra is demonstrated in its entirety, and the occipital base and mandibular mentum are (D) _____ .

---

4. How is the patient positioned for an AP cervical projection to prevent rotation of the upper and lower cervical vertebrae?

A. Upper: _____

_____

B. Lower: _____

_____

5. When the patient and cervical vertebrae are rotated away from the AP projection, the vertebral bodies will move

toward the side positioned (A) _____ (closer to/farther from) the IR, and the spinous processes will move

toward the side positioned (B) _____ (closer to/farther from) the IR.

6. Will rotation on an AP cervical projection with poor positioning always be demonstrated throughout the entire cervical column?

A. _____ (Yes/No)

Explain your answer.

B. _____

_____

7. A patient wearing a collar and on a backboard is taken to the radiography department for a cervical vertebrae series. Should the collar be removed before the radiographs are taken?

A. _____ (Yes/No)

The patient's head is rotated. Should it be adjusted?

B. _____ (Yes/No)

Explain your answers to parts A and B.

C. _____

_____

8. What is the curvature of the cervical vertebral column?

_____

9. How do the intervertebral disk spaces slant on the cervical vertebrae?

A. _____

Is the degree of slant higher when the patient is upright or supine?

B. _____

What CR angulation is used for an AP cervical projection in a supine patient?

C. _____

In an upright patient?

D. _____

What causes this difference?

E. _____

10. If the CR angulation is not adequately angled for an AP cervical projection, the intervertebral disk spaces are (A) _____, and each vertebra's spinous process is demonstrated within (B) _____ _____.

11. Where is each vertebra's spinous process demonstrated if the CR angulation is too cephalad?

    _____

12. Does too much or too little cephalad angulation cause elongation of the uncinate processes on an AP cervical projection? _____

13. How is the patient positioned to demonstrate the third cervical vertebra in its entirety on an AP cervical projection with accurate positioning? _____

    _____

14. Accurate CR centering on an AP cervical projection is obtained by placing the CR at the patient's (A) _____ plane at a level halfway between the (B) _____ and (C) _____.

15. Which anatomic structures are demonstrated on an AP cervical projection with accurate positioning? _____

    _____

For the following descriptions of AP cervical projections with poor positioning, state how the patient or CR would have been mispositioned for such a projection to be obtained.

16. The spinous processes are not aligned with the midline of the cervical bodies, and the pedicles and articular pillars are not symmetrically demonstrated lateral to the vertebral bodies. The right mandibular angle is visible, the left mandibular angle is superimposed over the cervical vertebrae, and the medial end of the right clavicle is demonstrated without vertebral column superimposition.

    _____

17. The anteroinferior aspects of the cervical bodies are obscuring the intervertebral disk spaces, and each vertebra's spinous process is demonstrated within the vertebral body.

    _____

18. The posteroinferior aspects of the cervical bodies are obscuring the intervertebral disk spaces, the uncinate processes are elongated, and each vertebra's spinous process is demonstrated within the inferior adjoining vertebral body.

    _____

19. A portion of the third cervical vertebra is superimposed over the occipital bone.

    _____

    _____

20. The mandibular mentum is superimposed over a portion of the third cervical vertebra.

    _____

21. The upper cervical vertebra is tilted toward the left side.

    _____

    _____

For the following AP cervical projections with poor positioning, state which anatomic structures are misaligned and how the patient should be repositioned for an optimal projection to be obtained.

Figure 8-3

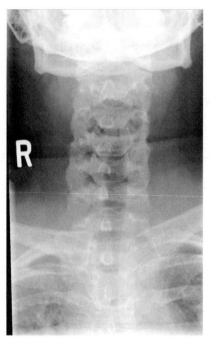

22. Figure 8-3: _____

_____

_____

_____

Figure 8-4

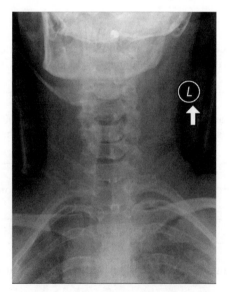

23. Figure 8-4: _____

_____

_____

_____

Figure 8-5

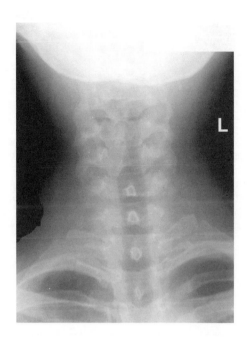

24. Figure 8-5: _____

_____

_____

_____

Figure 8-6

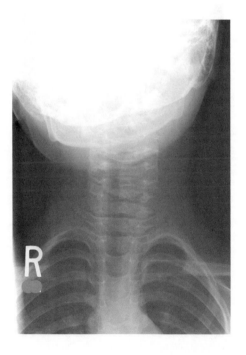

25. Figure 8-6: _____

_____

_____

_____

369

Figure 8-7

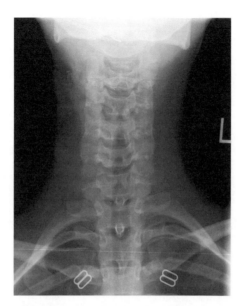

26. Figure 8-7: _____

_____

_____

_____

Figure 8-8

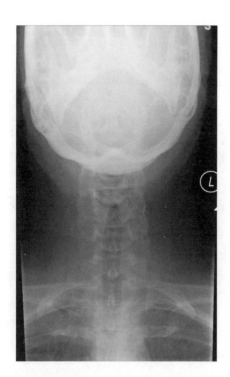

27. Figure 8-8: _____

_____

_____

_____

Figure 8-9

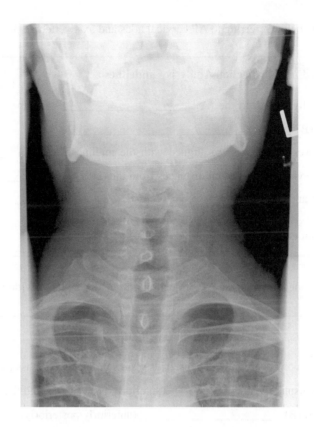

28. Figure 8-9: _____

_____

_____

_____

Cervical Atlas and Axis: AP Projection (Open Mouth)

29. Identify the labeled anatomy in Figure 8-10.

Figure 8-10

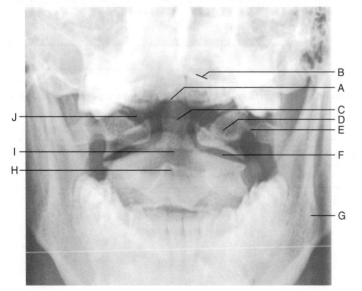

A. _____

B. _____

C. _____

D. _____

E. _____

F. _____

G. _____

H. _____

I. _____

J. _____

30. Complete the statements below referring to AP cervical atlas and axis vertebrae projection analysis guidelines.

AP Cervical Atlas and Axis Projection Analysis Guidelines

- Atlas is symmetrically seated on the (A) _____, with the atlas's lateral masses at equal distances from the (B) _____.
- The spinous processes of the axis are aligned with the midline of the (C) _____ body, and the mandibular rami are visualized at equal distances from the (D) _____.
- The upper incisors and the occipital base are seen (E) _____ to the dens and the atlantoaxial joint.
- The atlantoaxial joint is (F) _____.

---

31. How is the patient positioned to obtain an AP projection of the atlas and axis without rotation?

_____

_____

32. On head rotation, the atlas pivots around the dens. This results in the lateral mass located on the side toward which the face is turned being displaced (A) _____ (anteriorly/posteriorly), and the side away from which the face is turned being displaced (B) _____ (anteriorly/posteriorly).

33. How is the patient positioned for an AP projection of the atlas and axis to demonstrate the upper incisor and occipital base superior to the dens and atlantoaxial joint?

A. _____

_____

34. Why is it necessary to use a 5-degree cephalic CR angulation on an AP atlas and axis projection? _____

_____

35. Describe how to determine the CR angulation to use for an AP atlas and axis projection on a trauma patient in a collar.

_____

_____

36. How can one determine from a trauma AP atlas or axis projection that the CR angulation was too cephalic for the projection?

A. _____

That the CR was too caudal for the projection?

B. _____

37. Accurate CR centering on an AP atlas and axis projection is accomplished by centering the CR through the open mouth to the _____.

38. Which anatomic structures are included on an AP atlas and axis projection with accurate positioning?

_____

_____

For the following descriptions of AP atlas and axis cervical projections with poor positioning, state how the patient or CR would have been mispositioned for such a projection to be obtained.

39. The distances from the atlas's lateral masses to the dens and from the mandibular rami to the dens are narrower on the right side of the patient than on the left side, and the axis's spinous process is shifted from the midline.

_____

40. The upper incisors are demonstrated approximately 1 inch (2.5 cm) inferior to the occipital base, obscuring the dens and atlantoaxial joint, and the occipital base is demonstrated directly superior to the dens.

_____

41. The upper incisors are superimposed over the dens, and the occipital base is demonstrated superior to the dens and upper incisors. A 5-degree cephalic angulation was used to obtain this projection.

A. Patient: _____

_____

B. CR: _____

_____

42. The dens is superimposed over the occiput, and the upper incisors are demonstrated approximately 2 inches (5 cm) superior to the occipital base.

A. Patient: _____

_____

B. CR: _____

For the following AP atlas and axis cervical projections with poor positioning, state which anatomic structures are misaligned and how the patient should be repositioned for an optimal projection to be obtained.

Figure 8-11

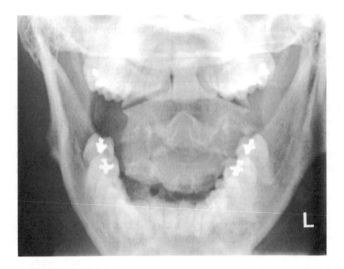

43. Figure 8-11: _____

_____

_____

_____

Figure 8-12

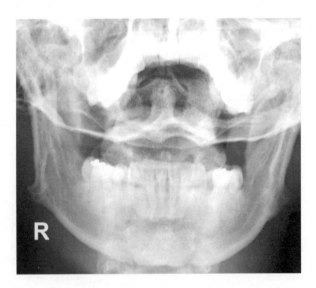

44. Figure 8-12: _____

_____

_____

_____

Figure 8-13

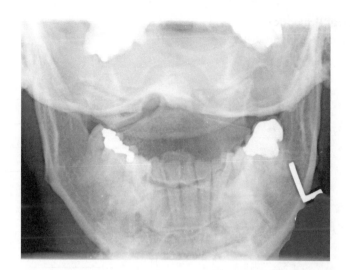

45. Figure 8-13: _____

_____

_____

_____

Figure 8-14

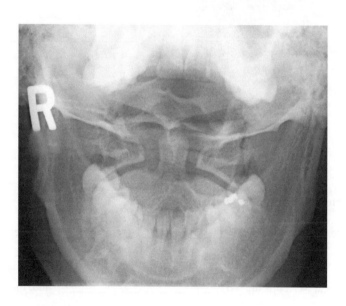

46. Figure 8-14 was taken with the patient in a cervical collar: _____

_____

_____

_____

Cervical Vertebrae: Lateral Projection

47. Identify the labeled anatomy in Figure 8-15.

Figure 8-15

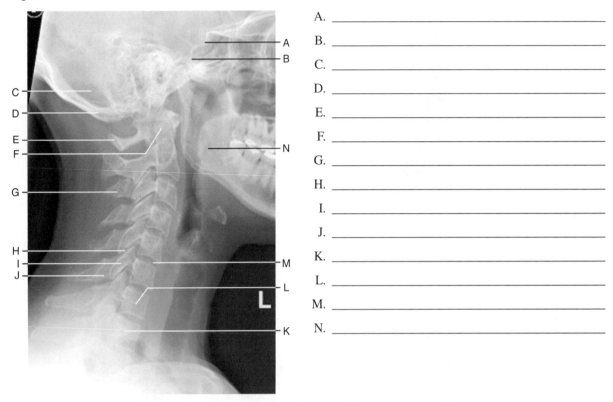

A. _____

B. _____

C. _____

D. _____

E. _____

F. _____

G. _____

H. _____

I. _____

J. _____

K. _____

L. _____

M. _____

N. _____

48. Complete the statements below referring to lateral cervical vertebrae projection analysis guidelines.

Lateral Cervical Vertebrae Projection Analysis Guidelines

■ Contrast is adequate to visualize the (A) _____ fat stripe.

■ The anterior and posterior aspects of the right and left articular pillars and the right and left zygapophyseal joints of each cervical vertebra are (B) _____, and the spinous processes are in

(C) _____.

■ The posterior arch of C1 and spinous process of C2 are in profile without (D) _____ obstruction, their bodies are seen without mandibular superimposition, the mandibular rami are

(E) _____, the superior and inferior aspects of the right and left articular pillars and the

(F) _____ of each cervical vertebra are superimposed, and the intervertebral disk spaces are open.

---

49. Which body plane is positioned perpendicular to the IR for a lateral cervical projection? _____

50. Which anatomic structures are aligned with the IR to prevent rotation when positioning the patient for a lateral cervical projection?

_____

51. How can rotation be identified on a lateral cervical projection with poor positioning?

_____

52. How must the patient's head be positioned for a lateral cervical projection to demonstrate the posterior arch of C1 and the spinous process of C2 in profile without occiput superimposition, and the bodies of C1 and C2 without mandibular rami superimposition?

_____

_____

53. How must the patient's head be positioned for a lateral cervical projection to superimpose the superior and inferior aspects of the right and left articular pillars and zygapophyseal joints?

_____

_____

54. Why are lateral flexion and extension projections of the cervical vertebrae obtained?

_____

55. How is patient positioning adjusted from a neutral lateral position of the cervical vertebrae to achieve a flexed lateral projection?

_____

_____

56. How is patient positioning adjusted from a neutral lateral position of the cervical vertebrae to achieve an extended lateral projection?

_____

_____

57. Accurate CR centering on a lateral cervical projection is accomplished by centering the CR to the (A) _____ plane at a level halfway between the (B) _____ and (C) _____.

58. Which anatomic structures are included on a lateral cervical projection with accurate positioning?

_____

_____

59. Why should the clivus be included on all lateral cervical projections?

_____

_____

60. It is often difficult to demonstrate C7 on a routine lateral cervical projection because of shoulder thickness. How should the patient be positioned to improve C7 demonstration?

A. _____

B. _____

C. _____

61. What special projection can be taken to demonstrate C7 when the procedures referred to in the previous question

fail? _____

For the following descriptions of lateral cervical projections with poor positioning, state how the patient would have been mispositioned for such a projection to be obtained.

62. The articular pillars and zygapophyseal joints of one side of the patient are situated anterior to the opposite side's pillars and zygapophyseal joints.

_____

63. Neither the posterior nor the anterior cortices of the cranium nor the mandible is superimposed.

_____

64. The inferior cortices of the cranium and mandible are demonstrated without superimposition, and the vertebral foramen of C1 is demonstrated.

_____

For the following lateral cervical projections with poor positioning, state which anatomic structures are misaligned and how the patient should be repositioned for an optimal projection to be obtained.

Figure 8-16

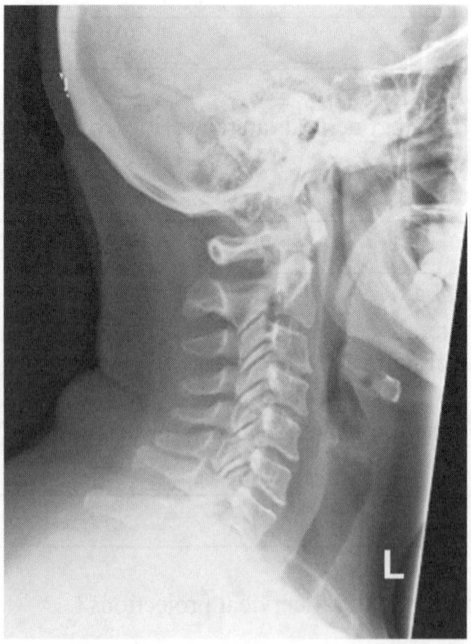

65. Figure 8-16: _____

_____

_____

_____

Figure 8-17

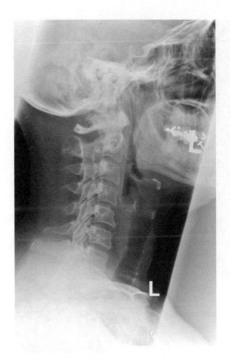

66. Figure 8-17: _____

_____

_____

_____

Figure 8-18

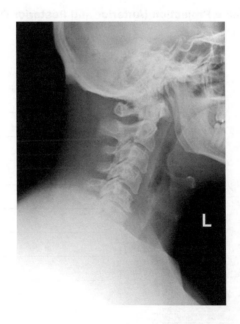

67. Figure 8-18: _____

_____

_____

_____

Figure 8-19

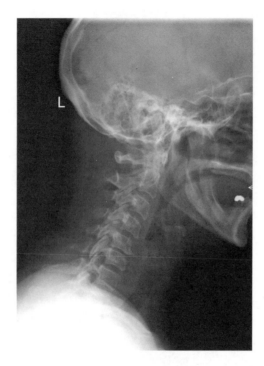

68. Figure 8-19: _____

_____

_____

_____

Cervical Vertebrae: PA/AP Axial Oblique Projection (Anterior and Posterior Oblique Positions)

69. Identify the labeled anatomy in Figure 8-20.

Figure 8-20

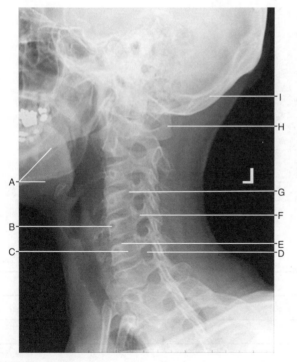

A. _____

B. _____

C. _____

D. _____

E. _____

F. _____

G. _____

H. _____

I. _____

70. Complete the statements below referring to PA/AP axial oblique cervical vertebrae projection analysis guidelines.

> **PA/AP Axial Oblique Cervical Vertebrae Projection Analysis Guidelines**
>
> - The second through (A) _____ intervertebral foramina are open, demonstrating uniform size and shape, the pedicles of interest are shown in (B) _____, and the opposite pedicles are aligned with the (C) _____ vertebral bodies.
> - The intervertebral disk spaces are open, the cervical bodies are seen as individual structures and are uniform in shape, and the posterior arch of the atlas is seen without foreshortening, demonstrating the
>
>   (D) _____.

71. For the following oblique cervical projections, state whether the right or left intervertebral foramina will be demonstrated.

    A. Right PA axial oblique (RAO position): _____

    B. Left AP axial oblique (LPO position): _____

    C. Left PA axial oblique (LAO position): _____

    D. Right AP axial oblique (RPO position): _____

72. What degree of body rotation is used for oblique cervical projections? _____

73. Which body plane is used to set up the degree of obliquity? _____

74. Describe how to position the IR beneath a trauma patient to demonstrate the right intervertebral foramina for an AP axial oblique cervical projection.

    A. _____

    How is the CR angled and positioned?

    B. _____

75. What degree and direction of CR angulation are used for PA axial oblique cervical projections?

    A. _____

    For AP axial oblique cervical projections?

    B. _____

    Why is it necessary to use an angled CR for oblique cervical projections?

    C. _____

76. How should the patient be positioned to demonstrate the alignment of the right and left posterior cranium and mandible cortices and to demonstrate the upper cervical vertebrae without occipital or mandibular superimposition?

    _____

    _____

77. How should the CR be adjusted from the routinely used angle for a PA axial oblique cervical vertebrae projection in a patient who has severe kyphosis to better demonstrate the lower cervical vertebrae?

    _____

    _____

78. Which cranial and mandibular cortices will be demonstrated inferiorly on a right PA axial oblique cervical projection?

A. _____

On a left AP axial oblique cervical projection?

B. _____

Which aspect of the positioning setup causes these cortices to be projected one superior to the other?

C. _____

_____

79. Accurate CR centering on a PA axial oblique cervical projection is accomplished by centering the CR to the

(A) _____ plane at a level halfway between the (B) _____ and

(C) _____ .

80. Which anatomic structures are included on PA/AP axial oblique cervical projections with accurate positioning?

_____

_____

_____

For the following descriptions of PA/AP axial oblique cervical projections with poor positioning, state how the patient or CR would have been mispositioned for such a projection to be obtained.

81. A left PA axial oblique (LAO) cervical projection, obtained with the patient's head in an oblique position, demonstrates obscured pedicles and intervertebral foramina, and the vertebral column is superimposed over a portion of the left sternoclavicular joint and medial clavicular end.

_____

82. A right PA axial oblique (RAO) cervical projection, obtained with the patient's head in a lateral position, demonstrates the intervertebral foramina, the right pedicles (although they are not in true profile), the left pedicles in the midline of the vertebral bodies, and the right zygapophyseal joints.

_____

83. A left PA axial oblique (LAO) cervical projection, the intervertebral disk spaces are closed, the vertebral bodies are distorted, the zygapophyseal joint spaces are demonstrated, the C1 vertebral foramen is not demonstrated, and the inferior mandibular rami and the cranial cortices are demonstrated with superimposition.

_____

84. The upper cervical vertebrae are obscured by the patient's cranium and mandible.

_____

85. A PA axial oblique with the atlas and its posterior arch are obscured. The inferior cranial cortices demonstrate more than 0.25 inch (0.6 cm) of distance between them, and the inferior cortices of the mandibular rami demonstrate more than 0.5 inch (1.25 cm) of distance between them.

_____

For the following PA/AP axial oblique cervical projections with poor positioning, state which anatomic structures are misaligned and how the patient should be repositioned for such a projection to be obtained.

Figure 8-21

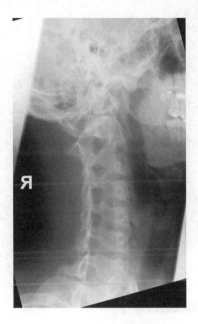

86. Figure 8-21: _____

_____

_____

_____

_____

_____

Figure 8-22

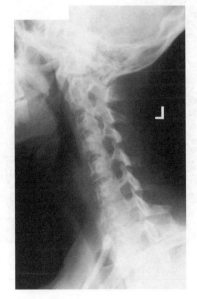

87. Figure 8-22: _____

_____

_____

Figure 8-23

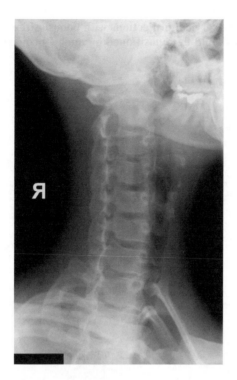

88. Figure 8-23: _____

_____

_____

Figure 8-24

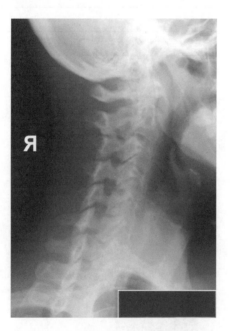

89. Figure 8-24: _____

_____

_____

Figure 8-25

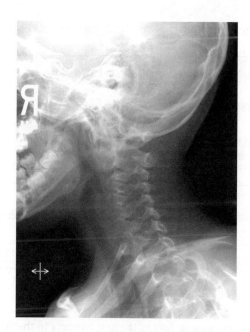

90. Figure 8-25: _____

_____

_____

_____

Cervicothoracic Vertebrae: Lateral Projection (Swimmer's Technique)

91. Identify the labeled anatomy in Figure 8-26.

Figure 8-26

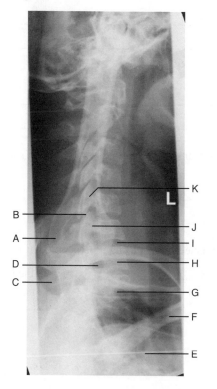

A. _____

B. _____

C. _____

D. _____

E. _____

F. _____

G. _____

H. _____

I. _____

J. _____

K. _____

92. Complete the statements below referring to lateral cervicothoracic vertebrae projection analysis guidelines.

Lateral Cervicothoracic Vertebrae Projection Analysis Guidelines

■ The right and left cervical zygapophyseal joints, the (A) _____, and the posterior ribs are superimposed.

■ The humerus elevated above the patient's head is aligned with the (B) _____.

■ The intervertebral disk spaces are (C) _____.

---

93. List two situations in which a cervicothoracic lateral projection would be indicated.

A. _____

B. _____

94. What respiration is used for the cervicothoracic lateral projection? _____

95. To obtain a cervicothoracic lateral projection, how is the arm adjacent to the IR positioned?

A. _____

How is the arm situated farther from the IR positioned?

B. _____

96. How is the patient positioned to prevent rotation on a lateral cervicothoracic projection?

A. Cervical rotation: _____

_____

B. Thoracic rotation: _____

_____

97. How can rotation be identified on a lateral cervicothoracic projection?

_____

_____

98. How is the patient positioned for a lateral cervicothoracic projection to demonstrate open intervertebral disk spaces and undistorted vertebral bodies?

_____

_____

99. Accurate CR centering on a lateral cervicothoracic projection is accomplished by centering a perpendicular CR to

the (A) _____ plane at a level 1 inch (2.5 cm) superior to the (B) _____ or at the level

of the (C) _____.

100. When should a 5-degree caudal CR angulation be used with the cervicothoracic lateral projection?

_____

101. Which anatomic structures are included on a lateral cervicothoracic projection with accurate positioning?

_____

For the following descriptions of lateral cervicothoracic projections with poor positioning, state how the patient would have been mispositioned for such a projection to be obtained.

102. The right and left articular pillars, zygapophyseal joints, and posterior ribs are demonstrated without superimposition. The humerus that was raised and situated closer to the IR is demonstrated posterior to the vertebral column.

_____

103. The right and left articular pillars, zygapophyseal joints, and posterior ribs are demonstrated without superimposition. The humerus demonstrating the lesser amount of magnification is situated anterior to the vertebral column.

_____

104. The intervertebral disk spaces are closed, and the vertebral bodies are distorted.

_____

For the following lateral cervicothoracic projections with poor positioning, state which anatomic structures are misaligned and how the patient should be repositioned for an optimal projection to be obtained.

Figure 8-27

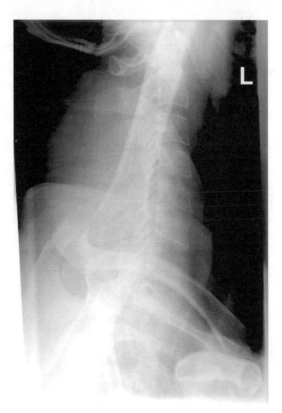

105. Figure 8-27: _____

_____

_____

Chapter **8 Image Analysis of the Cervical and Thoracic Vertebrae**

Figure 8-28

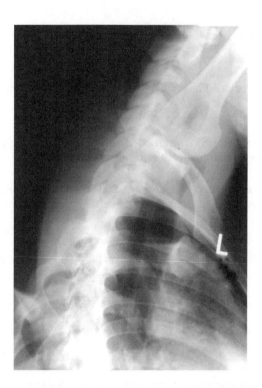

106. Figure 8-28: _____

_____

_____

Thoracic Vertebrae: AP Projection

107. Identify the labeled anatomy in Figure 8-29.

Figure 8-29

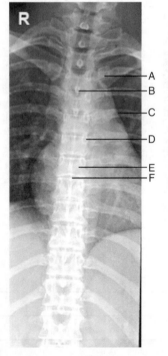

A. _____

B. _____

C. _____

D. _____

E. _____

F. _____

108. Complete the statements below referring to AP thoracic vertebrae projection analysis guidelines.

AP Thoracic Vertebrae Projection Analysis Guidelines

- The spinous processes are aligned with the midline of the (A) _____, and the distances from the vertebral column to the sternal clavicular ends and from the pedicles to the (B) _____ _____ are equal on the two sides.
- The intervertebral disk spaces are (C) _____, and the vertebral bodies are seen without foreshortening.

---

109. How tightly can one safely collimate transversely on an AP projection of the thoracic vertebrae?

_____

110. How can the patient be positioned with respect to the x-ray tube for an AP thoracic projection to take advantage of the anode-heel effect?

_____

_____

111. Which patient respiration is used for an AP thoracic projection to demonstrate the vertebrae and posterior ribs?

_____

112. How is the patient positioned to ensure that rotation will not be demonstrated on an AP thoracic projection?

_____

_____

113. When rotation is present on an AP thoracic projection, the side demonstrating the greater distance between the spinous processes and pedicles will be _____ (closer to/farther from) the IR.

114. Which patient condition can simulate rotation on an AP thoracic projection?

A. _____

Describe how this condition can be distinguished from rotation.

B. _____

_____

115. What type of curvature does the thoracic vertebral column demonstrate?

A. _____

How can the patient be positioned to reduce this curvature and better align the x-ray beams with the intervertebral disk spaces?

B. _____

_____

Chapter **8 Image Analysis of the Cervical and Thoracic Vertebrae**

116. Accurate CR centering on an AP thoracic projection is accomplished by centering the CR to the (A) _____ plane at a level halfway between the (B) _____ and the xiphoid.

117. Which anatomic structures are included on an AP thoracic projection with accurate positioning?

_____

For the following descriptions of AP thoracic projections with poor positioning, state how the patient would have been mispositioned for such a projection to be obtained.

118. The lower thoracic intervertebral disk spaces are obscured, and the vertebral bodies are distorted.

_____

119. The distance from the left pedicles to the spinous processes is greater than the distance from the right pedicles to the spinous processes.

_____

120. The upper thoracic vertebrae are overexposed, and the lower thoracic vertebrae demonstrate adequate brightness.

_____

For the following AP thoracic projections with poor positioning, state which anatomic structures are misaligned and how the patient should be repositioned for an optimal projection to be obtained.

Figure 8-30

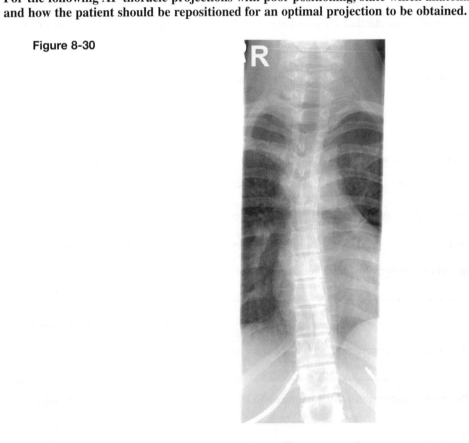

121. Figure 8-30: _____

_____

_____

Figure 8-31

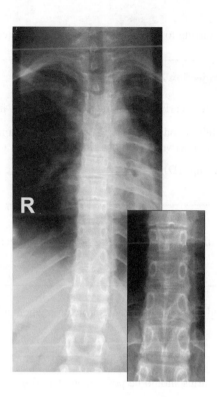

122. Figure 8-31: _____

_____

Thoracic Vertebrae: Lateral Projection

123. Identify the labeled anatomy in Figure 8-32.

Figure 8-32

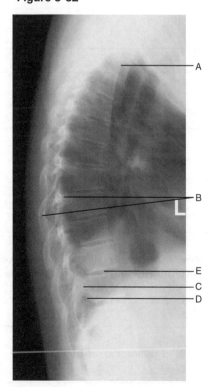

A. _____

B. _____

C. _____

D. _____

E. _____

124. Complete the statements below referring to lateral thoracic vertebrae projection analysis guidelines.

Lateral Thoracic Vertebrae Projection Analysis Guidelines
■ The intervertebral foramina are clearly demonstrated, pedicles are in (A) _____, the posterior surfaces of each vertebral body are (B) _____, and no more than (C) _____ inch(es) of space is demonstrated between the posterior ribs.
■ The intervertebral disk spaces are (D) _____, and the vertebral bodies are demonstrated without distortion.

125. What advantage does using a breathing technique over a nonbreathing technique have when imaging the thoracic vertebrae in the lateral projection?

_____

126. If patient motion cannot be avoided on a lateral thoracic projection when using a breathing technique, what respiration should be used?

_____

127. List two reasons why the patient's arms should be positioned at a 90-degree angle with the body for a lateral thoracic projection.

A. _____

_____

B. _____

_____

128. How is the patient positioned to prevent rotation on a lateral thoracic projection?

_____

_____

129. How can rotation be identified on a lateral thoracic projection?

_____

_____

130. How can scoliosis be distinguished from rotation on a lateral thoracic projection?

_____

_____

131. When the thoracic vertebrae are in a lateral projection, the posterior surfaces of the vertebral bodies are positioned on top of each other. Why does the resulting projection demonstrate the posterior ribs without superimposition?

_____

_____

132. How is the patient positioned to obtain open intervertebral disk spaces on a lateral thoracic projection?

_____

133. Describe the patient body forms that demonstrate the greatest thoracic vertebral sagging when the patient is placed in a lateral projection.

   A. _____

   B. _____

State where the radiolucent sponge is positioned to offset this sagging.

   C. _____

State how the CR can be adjusted to offset this sagging.

   D. _____

134. Accurate CR centering on a lateral thoracic vertebral projection is accomplished by centering the CR to the _____ when the patient's arm is positioned at a 90-degree angle with the body.

135. Which anatomic structures are included on a lateral thoracic projection with accurate positioning?

   _____

136. List two methods of confirming which thoracic vertebra is the 12th on a lateral thoracic projection.

   A. _____

   B. _____

   _____

137. List two methods of confirming which thoracic vertebra is the first on a lateral thoracic projection.

   A. _____

   B. _____

138. If the first, second, or third thoracic vertebra is not included on a routine lateral thoracic projection, which supplementary projection is used to demonstrate these vertebrae?

For the following descriptions of lateral thoracic projections with poor positioning, state how the patient would have been mispositioned for such a projection to be obtained.

139. The posterior surfaces of the vertebral bodies are demonstrated without superimposition, and more than 0.5 inch (1.25 cm) of space is demonstrated between the posterior ribs.

   _____

140. The posterior surfaces of the vertebral bodies are demonstrated without superimposition, and the posterior ribs are superimposed.

   _____

141. The 8th through 12th thoracic intervertebral disk spaces are obscured, and the vertebral bodies are distorted.

   _____

For the following lateral thoracic projections with poor positioning, state which anatomic structures are misaligned and how the patient should be repositioned for an optimal projection to be obtained.

Figure 8-33

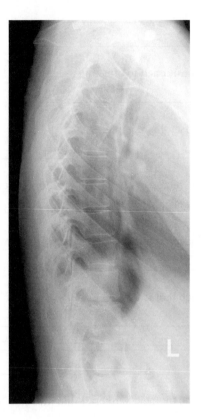

142. Figure 8-33: _____

_____

_____

Figure 8-34

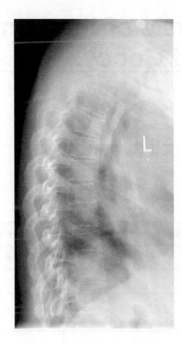

143. Figure 8-34: _____

_____

_____

_____

_____

Figure 8-35

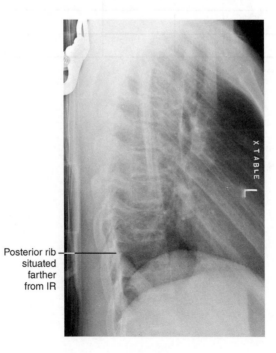

Posterior rib situated farther from IR

144. Figure 8-35, cross-table trauma projection: _____

_____

_____

Chapter **8 Image Analysis of the Cervical and Thoracic Vertebrae**

Image Analysis of the Lumbar Vertebrae, Sacrum, and Coccyx

STUDY QUESTIONS

1. Complete Figure 9-1.

Figure 9-1

Lumbar Vertebrae, Sacrum, and Coccyx Technical Data					
Projection	kV	Grid	AEC	mAs	SID
AP, lumber vertebrae					
AP oblique, lumbar vertebrae					
Lateral, lumbar vertebrae					
Lateral, L5-S1 lumbosacral junction					
AP axial, sacrum					
Lateral, sacrum					
AP axial, coccyx					
Lateral, coccyx					
Pediatric					

Lumbar Vertebrae: AP Projection

2. Identify the labeled anatomy in Figure 9-2.

Figure 9-2

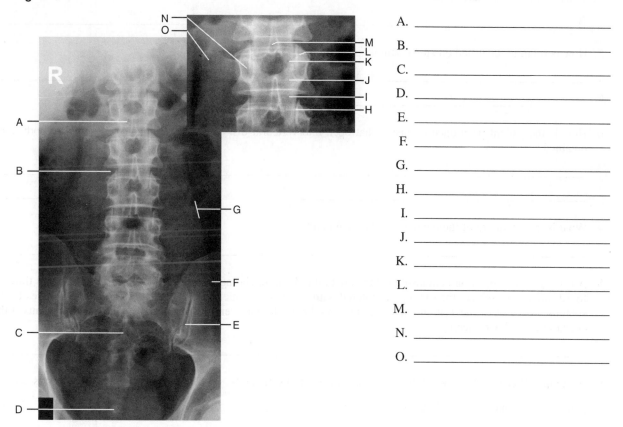

A. _____

B. _____

C. _____

D. _____

E. _____

F. _____

G. _____

H. _____

I. _____

J. _____

K. _____

L. _____

M. _____

N. _____

O. _____

3. Complete the statements below referring to AP lumbar vertebrae projection analysis guidelines.

AP Lumbar Vertebrae Projection Analysis Guidelines

- The distances from the pedicles to the (A) _____ are (B) _____ on both sides. The sacrum and coccyx should be centered within the inlet pelvis and aligned with the pubis symphysis.

- The intervertebral disk spaces are (C) _____, and the vertebral bodies are seen without distortion.

- The (D) _____ are aligned with the midline of the vertebral bodies.

---

4. Which soft tissue structures are to be included on an AP lumbar projection?

   A. _____

   Where are these structures located?

   B. _____

5. How is rotation identified on an AP lumbar projection?

   _____

   _____

6. How is the patient positioned to ensure that open intervertebral disk spaces and undistorted vertebral bodies are obtained?

   _____

   _____

7. What is the curvature of the lumbar vertebral column?

   _____

8. An AP lumbar projection demonstrates the vertebral column deviating laterally at the level of the second through fourth lumbar vertebrae, the sacrum is centered within the pelvic inlet, and the distances from the pedicles to the spinous processes of the 11th thoracic vertebra and the 5th lumbar vertebra are nearly equal. What has caused the appearance of this projection?

   _____

9. Accurate CR centering on an AP lumbar projection taken using an 8- × 14-inch (20- × 35-cm) field size is accomplished by centering the CR to the (A) _____ plane at a level 1.5 inches (4 cm) (B) _____ to the (C) _____.

10. Which anatomic structures are included on an AP lumbar projection with accurate positioning taken using an 8- × 14-inch (20- × 35-cm) field size?

    _____

11. Accurate CR centering on an AP lumbar projection taken using an 8- × 17-inch (20- × 43-cm) field size is accomplished by centering the CR to the (A) _____ plane at the level of the (B) _____.

12. Which anatomic structures are included on an AP lumbar projection with accurate positioning taken using an 8- × 17-inch (20- × 43-cm) field size?

    _____

13. How tightly can the transversely collimated field be coned and still include all the required anatomic structures?

    _____

For the following descriptions of AP lumbar projections with poor positioning, state how the patient would have been mispositioned for such a projection to be obtained.

14. The distance from the right pedicles to the spinous processes is less than the distance from the left pedicles to the spinous processes, and the sacrum and coccyx are rotated toward the right lateral inlet pelvis.

    _____

15. The first through third lumbar vertebrae are demonstrated without rotation, the fourth and fifth vertebrae are rotated, and the sacrum and coccyx are rotated toward the patient's left side.

_____

16. The intervertebral disk spaces between the 12th thoracic vertebra and the 3rd lumbar vertebra are closed, and these lumbar bodies are distorted. The iliac spines are demonstrated without pelvic brim superimposition.

_____

For the following AP lumbar projections with poor positioning, state which anatomic structures are misaligned and how the patient should be repositioned for an optimal projection to be obtained.

Figure 9-3

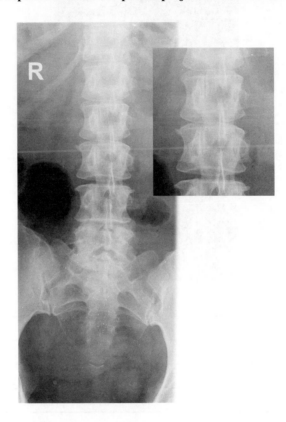

17. Figure 9-3: _____

_____

_____

Chapter **9** **Image Analysis of the Lumbar Vertebrae, Sacrum, and Coccyx**

Figure 9-4

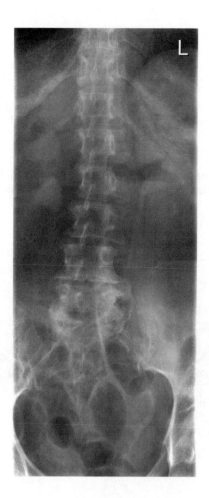

18. Figure 9-4: _____

_____

_____

_____

_____

_____

Figure 9-5

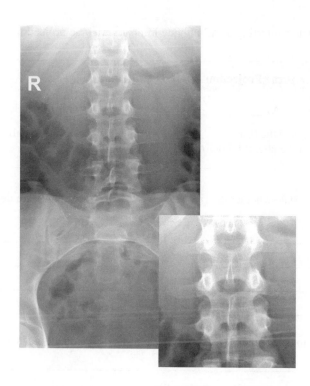

19. Figure 9-5: _____

_____

Lumbar Vertebrae: AP Oblique Projection (RPO and LPO Positions)

20. Identify the labeled anatomy in Figure 9-6.

Figure 9-6

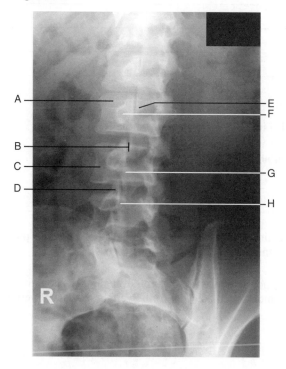

A. _____

B. _____

C. _____

D. _____

E. _____

F. _____

G. _____

H. _____

21. Complete the statements below referring to AP oblique lumbar vertebrae projection analysis guidelines.

AP Oblique Lumbar Vertebrae Projection Analysis Guidelines
■ The superior and inferior (A) _____ are in profile, the (B) _____ joints are demonstrated, and the (C) _____ are seen halfway between the midpoint of the vertebral bodies and the lateral border of the vertebral bodies.

22. For the following positions, state whether the right or left zygapophyseal joints are demonstrated on an AP oblique lumbar projection.

    A. RAO: _____

    B. LPO: _____

    C. RPO: _____

    D. LAO: _____

23. Which body plane is used to determine patient obliquity for an AP oblique lumbar projection?

    A. _____

    How much is the patient's torso rotated for an AP oblique lumbar projection?

    B. _____

24. Name the anatomic structures of the lumbar vertebrae that correspond with the parts of the "Scottie dog" listed below.

    A. Ear: _____

    B. Nose: _____

    C. Body: _____

    D. Eye: _____

    E. Front leg: _____

25. Accurate CR centering on an AP oblique lumbar projection is accomplished by centering the CR 2 inches (5 cm)

    (A) _____ to the elevated (B) _____ at a level 1.5 inches (4 cm) superior to the (C) _____.

26. Which anatomic structures are included on an AP oblique lumbar projection with accurate positioning?

    _____

    _____

For the following descriptions of AP oblique lumbar projections with poor positioning, state how the patient would have been mispositioned for such a projection to be obtained.

27. The vertebrae's superior and inferior articular processes are not demonstrated in profile, their corresponding zygapophyseal joint spaces are closed, and their pedicles are demonstrated adjacent to the vertebrae's lateral vertebral body borders.

    _____

    _____

28. The vertebrae's superior and inferior articular processes are not demonstrated in profile, their corresponding zygapophyseal joint spaces are closed, their laminae are obscured, and their pedicles are shown at the midpoint of the vertebral bodies.

For the following oblique lumbar projections with poor positioning, state which anatomic structures are misaligned and how the patient should be repositioned for an optimal projection to be obtained.

Figure 9-7

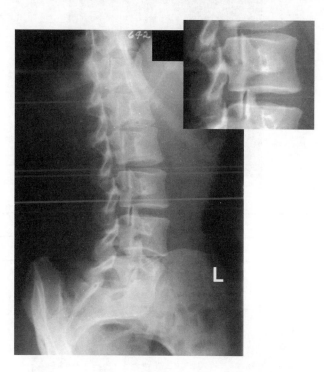

29. Figure 9-7: _____

_____

_____

Chapter **9 Image Analysis of the Lumbar Vertebrae, Sacrum, and Coccyx**

Figure 9-8

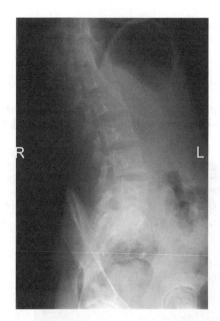

30. Figure 9-8: _____

_____

_____

Figure 9-9

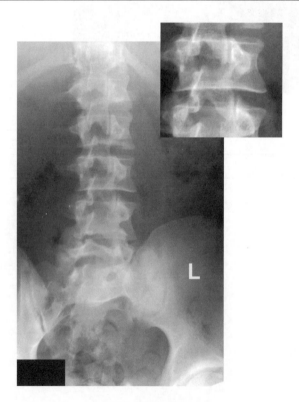

31. Figure 9-9: _____

_____

_____

Lumbar Vertebrae: Lateral Projection

32. Identify the labeled anatomy in Figure 9-10.

Figure 9-10

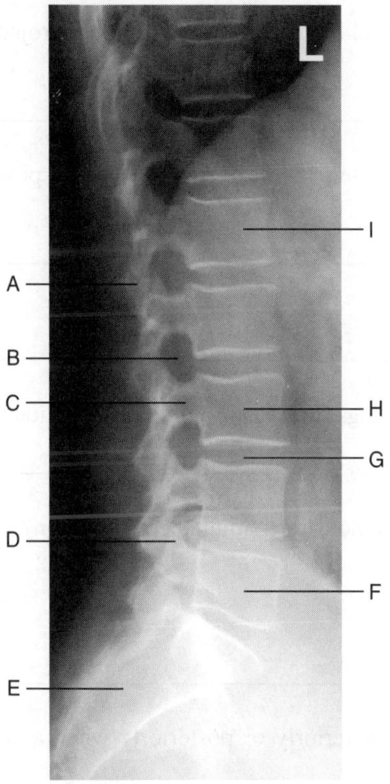

A. _____

B. _____

C. _____

D. _____

E. _____

F. _____

G. _____

H. _____

I. _____

33. Complete the statements below referring to lateral lumbar vertebrae projection analysis guidelines.

Lateral Lumbar Vertebrae Projection Analysis Guidelines

- The intervertebral foramina are demonstrated, and the (A) _____ are in profile.

- The right and left pedicles and the posterior surfaces of each vertebral body are (B) _____.

- The intervertebral disk spaces are (C) _____.

- The lumbar vertebral column is in a (D) _____ position without anteroposterior flexion or extension.

---

34. How is the patient positioned to prevent rotation on a lateral lumbar projection?

_____

_____

35. How is the patient positioned to ensure open intervertebral disk spaces and undistorted vertebral bodies on a lateral lumbar projection?

_____

36. Lumbar column lateral flexion or tilt with the IR most often occurs with which patient body types?

    A. _____

    B. _____

37. How can CR be adjusted to obtain open disk spaces and undistorted vertebral bodies on a lateral lumbar projection when the patient's vertebral column is tilted?

    _____

38. For a lateral lumbar projection, the patient may be placed on the imaging table in a left or right recumbent position unless the patient has which spinal condition?

    A. _____

    For this condition, how are the CR and vertebral column positioned?

    B. _____

39. What is accomplished by placing a pillow or sponge between the patient's legs for a lateral lumbar projection?

    _____

40. Will the upper and lower vertebrae on a lateral lumbar projection always demonstrate simultaneous rotation?

    A. _____ (Yes/No)

    Explain your answer.

    B. _____

41. Why is it difficult to determine which side of the body has been rotated anteriorly or posteriorly when a lateral lumbar projection demonstrates rotation?

    _____

42. Why are flexion and extension lateral lumbar projections requested?

    _____

43. Describe how patient positioning is adjusted from a neutral lateral position to place the patient in maximum flexion for a lateral lumbar projection.

    A. _____

    Describe how patient positioning is adjusted from a neutral lateral position to place the patient in maximum extension for a lateral lumbar projection.

    B. _____

44. The lordotic curvature on a lumbar projection is (A) _____ (increased/decreased) when the patient is positioned in maximum flexion and is (B) _____ (increased/decreased) when the patient is positioned in maximum extension.

45. Accurate CR centering on a lateral lumbar projection when an 8- × 14-inch (20- × 35-cm) field size is used is accomplished by centering the CR to the (A) _____ plane located halfway between the elevated (B) _____ and (C) _____ at a level 1.5 inches (4 cm) superior to the (D) _____.

46. Which anatomic structures are included on a lateral lumbar projection with accurate positioning taken on an 8- × 14-inch (20- × 35-cm) field size?

_____

47. Accurate CR centering on a lateral lumbar projection when an 8- × 17-inch (20- × 43-cm) field size is used is accomplished by centering the CR to the (A) _____ plane located halfway between the elevated (B) _____ and (C) _____ at the level of the (D) _____.

48. Which anatomic structures are included on a lateral lumbar projection with accurate positioning taken on an 8- × 17-inch (20- × 43-cm) field size?

_____

49. Describe two situations in which a tightly collimated lateral view of the L5-S1 lumbar region is indicated after the lateral lumbar projection has been reviewed.

   A. _____

   B. _____

For the following descriptions of lateral lumbar projections with poor positioning, state how the patient would have been mispositioned for such a projection to be obtained.

50. The posterior surfaces of the first through fourth vertebral bodies and the posterior ribs are demonstrated without superimposition. The most magnified ribs are demonstrated anteriorly.

_____

51. The L4-L5 and L5-S1 intervertebral disk spaces are closed, and the third through fifth vertebral bodies are distorted.

_____

52. Explain why the intervertebral joint spaces are closed on the lateral lumbar projection in Figure 9-11 even though the iliac crests and alae are perfectly superimposed.

Figure 9-11

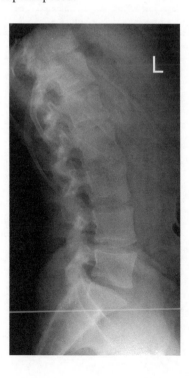

Chapter **9 Image Analysis of the Lumbar Vertebrae, Sacrum, and Coccyx**

For the following lateral lumbar projections with poor positioning, state which anatomic structures are misaligned and how the patient should be repositioned for an optimal projection to be obtained.

Figure 9-12

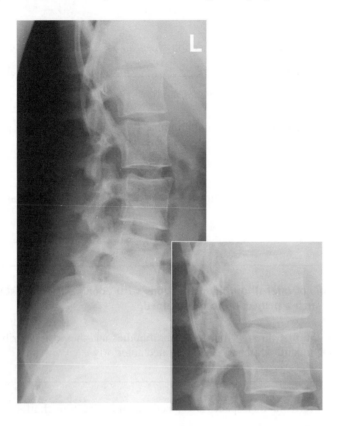

53. Figure 9-12: _____

_____

_____

_____

_____

Figure 9-13

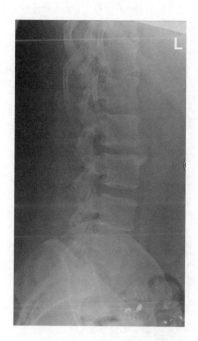

54. Figure 9-13: _____

_____

_____

Figure 9-14

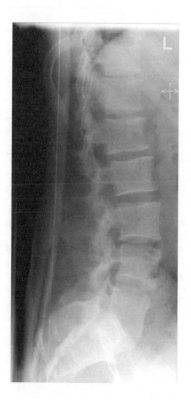

55. Figure 9-14: _____

_____

_____

Figure 9-15

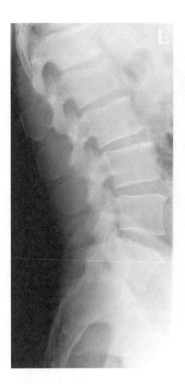

56. Figure 9-15: _____

_____

_____

L5-S1 Lumbosacral Junction: Lateral Projection
57. Identify the labeled anatomy in Figure 9-16.

Figure 9-16

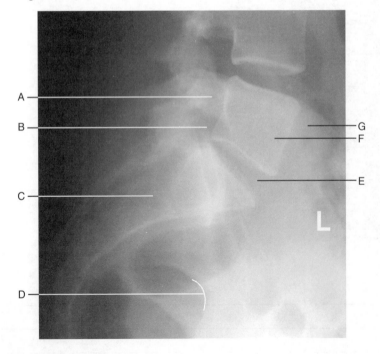

A. _____

B. _____

C. _____

D. _____

E. _____

F. _____

G. _____

Chapter **9 Image Analysis of the Lumbar Vertebrae, Sacrum, and Coccyx**

58. Complete the statements below referring to lateral L5-S1 lumbosacral junction projection analysis guidelines.

Lateral L5-S1 Lumbosacral Junction Projection Analysis Guidelines
■ The L5-S1 intervertebral foramen is demonstrated, the right and left (A) _____ are superimposed and in profile, and the (B) _____ are nearly superimposed.
■ The L5-S1 intervertebral disk space is (C) _____, the pelvic alae are nearly superimposed, and the sacrum is seen without distortion.

59. How tightly can the transverse field be collimated and still include the needed anatomic information on a lateral L5-S1 projection?

_____

60. What is accomplished by placing a pillow or sponge between the patient's legs for a lateral L5-S1 projection?

_____

_____

61. How can rotation be detected on a rotated lateral L5-S1 projection?

_____

_____

62. How is the patient positioned to obtain open intervertebral disk spaces and undistorted vertebral bodies on a lateral L5-S1 projection?

_____

63. How should the CR be adjusted to obtain an open L5-S1 joint space in a patient whose vertebral column curves upwardly?

_____

64. Accurate CR centering on a lateral L5-S1 projection is accomplished by centering the CR to a point 2 inches (5 cm) (A) _____ to the elevated (B) _____ and 1.5 inches (4 cm) (C) _____ to the (D) _____ _____.

65. Which anatomic structures are included on a lateral L5-S1 projection with accurate positioning?

_____

For the following descriptions of lateral L5-S1 lumbar projections with poor positioning, state how the patient would have been mispositioned for such a projection to be obtained.

66. The L5-S1 intervertebral foramen is obscured, and the greater sciatic notches and femoral heads are not superimposed.

_____

67. The L5-S1 intervertebral disk space is closed, and the pelvic alae are not superimposed.

_____

For the following lateral L5-S1 lumbar projections with poor positioning, state which anatomic structures are misaligned and how the patient should be repositioned for an optimal projection to be obtained.

Figure 9-17

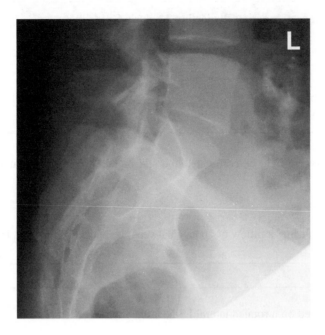

68. Figure 9-17: _____

_____

_____

Figure 9-18

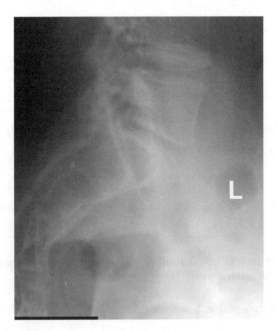

69. Figure 9-18: _____

_____

_____

412

Sacrum: AP Axial Projection

70. Identify the labeled anatomy in Figure 9-19.

Figure 9-19

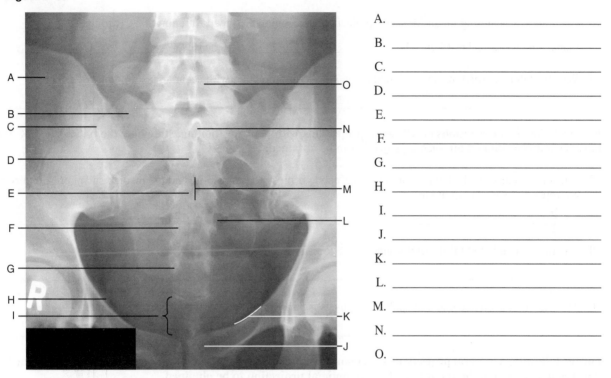

A. _____

B. _____

C. _____

D. _____

E. _____

F. _____

G. _____

H. _____

I. _____

J. _____

K. _____

L. _____

M. _____

N. _____

O. _____

71. Complete the statements below referring to AP axial sacrum projection analysis guidelines.

AP Axial Sacrum Projection Analysis Guidelines
■ The ischial spines are equally demonstrated and are aligned with the (A) _____, and the median sacral crest and (B) _____ are aligned with the pubis symphysis.
■ The first through (C) _____ sacral segments are seen without foreshortening, sacral foramina demonstrate equal spacing, and the (D) _____ is not superimposed over any portion of the sacrum.

72. Why is the patient instructed to empty the bladder and colon before an AP sacral projection is taken?

_____

_____

73. When a patient is rotated for an AP sacral projection, the sacrum rotates in the (A) _____ (opposite/same) direction as the pubis symphysis and is positioned next to the lateral pelvic brim situated (B) _____ (closer to/farther from) the IR.

74. What is the curvature of the sacrum? _____

413

75. How must the patient and CR be positioned to demonstrate the sacrum without foreshortening?

_____

_____

76. Accurate CR centering on an AP sacral projection is accomplished by positioning the CR to the (A) _____

plane at a level 2 inches (5 cm) (B) _____ to the (C) _____.

77. Which anatomic structures are included on an AP sacral projection with accurate positioning?

_____

For the following descriptions of AP sacral projections with poor positioning, state how the patient or CR would have been mispositioned for such a projection to be obtained.

78. The left ischial spine is demonstrated without pelvic brim superimposition, and the median sacral crest and coccyx are rotated toward the right hip.

_____

79. The first, second, and third sacral segments are foreshortened.

_____

80. The sacrum is elongated, and the pubis symphysis is superimposed over the fifth sacral segment.

_____

For the following AP sacral projections with poor positioning, state which anatomic structures are misaligned and how the patient should be repositioned for an optimal projection to be obtained.

Figure 9-20

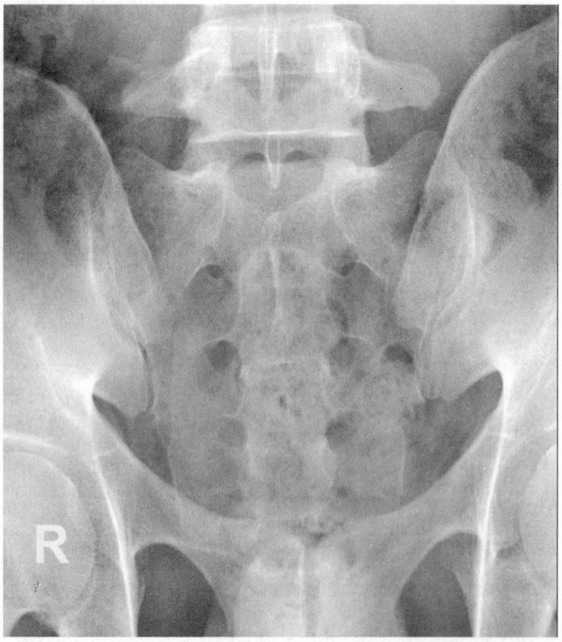

81. Figure 9-20: _____

_____

_____

414

Figure 9-21

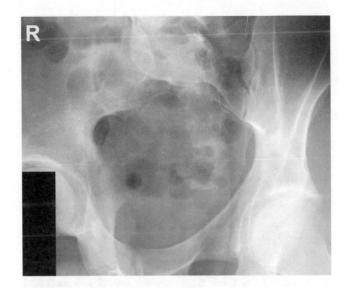

82. Figure 9-21: _____

_____

_____

_____

Figure 9-22

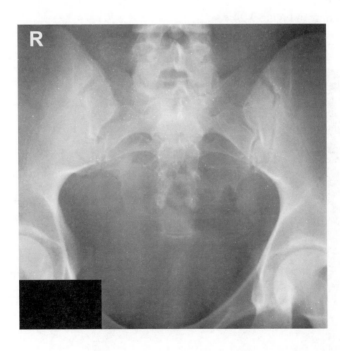

83. Figure 9-22: _____

_____

_____

_____

Chapter **9 Image Analysis of the Lumbar Vertebrae, Sacrum, and Coccyx**

Figure 9-23

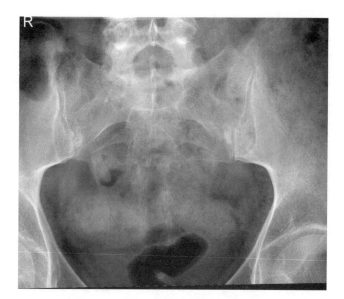

84. Figure 9-23: _____

_____

_____

Sacrum: Lateral Projection

85. Identify the labeled anatomy in Figure 9-24.

Figure 9-24

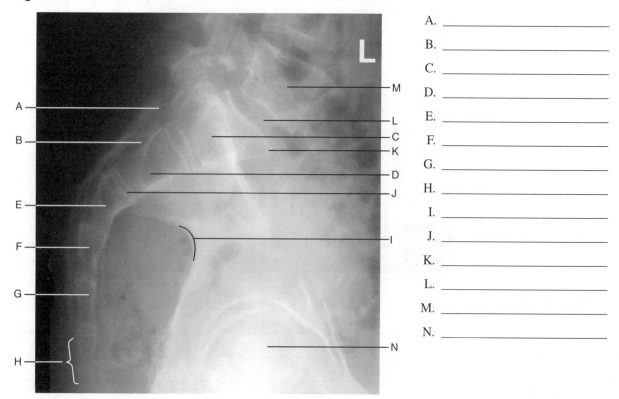

A. _____

B. _____

C. _____

D. _____

E. _____

F. _____

G. _____

H. _____

I. _____

J. _____

K. _____

L. _____

M. _____

N. _____

86. Complete the statements below referring to lateral sacrum projection analysis guidelines.

> **Lateral Sacrum Projection Analysis Guidelines**
>
> - The median sacral crest is in (A) _____, and the greater sciatic notches and the
>   (B) _____ are nearly superimposed.
> - The L5-S1 intervertebral disk space is open, pelvic alae are nearly (C) _____, and
>   the sacrum is seen without foreshortening.

87. How can rotation be detected on a rotated lateral sacral projection?

_____

_____

88. When a lateral sacral projection demonstrates rotation and the femoral heads are demonstrated on the projection, the

hip that is projected inferiorly is situated _____ (closer to/farther from) the IR.

89. How is the patient positioned to obtain an open L5-S1 disk space and an undistorted fifth lumbar body on a lateral
sacral projection?

_____

_____

90. How should the CR be adjusted to obtain an open L5-S1 intervertebral joint space in a patient whose vertebral
column curves upwardly?

_____

91. Accurate CR centering on a lateral sacral projection is accomplished by centering the CR to the (A) _____

plane located 3 to 4 inches (7.5 to 10 cm) posterior to the elevated (B) _____.

92. Which anatomic structures are included on a lateral sacral projection with accurate positioning?

_____

_____

**For the following descriptions of lateral sacral projections with poor positioning, state how the patient would have
been mispositioned for such a projection to be obtained.**

93. The greater sciatic notches are demonstrated without superimposition, the median sacral crest is not in profile, and
the inferiorly located femoral head is rotated posteriorly.

_____

94. The L5-S1 intervertebral disk space is closed, the fifth lumbar vertebra and sacrum are foreshortened, and the greater
sciatic notches are demonstrated without superimposition.

_____

Chapter **9 Image Analysis of the Lumbar Vertebrae, Sacrum, and Coccyx**

For the following lateral sacral projections with poor positioning, state which anatomic structures are misaligned and how the patient should be repositioned for an optimal projection to be obtained.

Figure 9-25

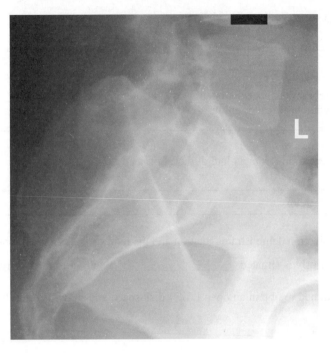

95. Figure 9-25: _____

_____

_____

Figure 9-26

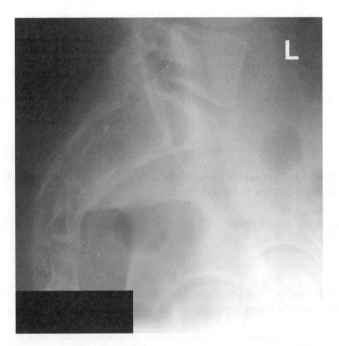

96. Figure 9-26:_____

_____

_____

Figure 9-27

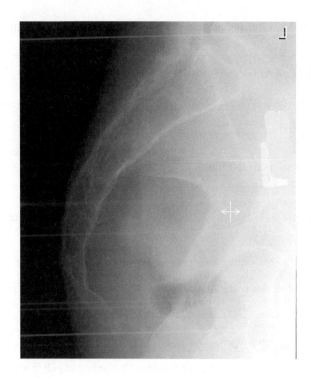

97. Figure 9-27: _____

_____

_____

Coccyx: AP Axial Projection

98. Identify the labeled anatomy in Figure 9-28.

Figure 9-28

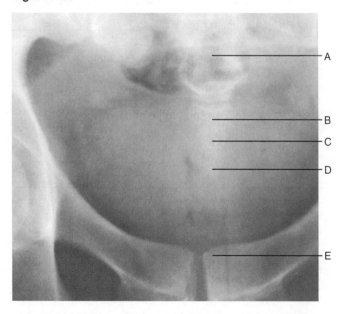

A. _____

B. _____

C. _____

D. _____

E. _____

99. Complete the statements below referring to AP axial coccyx projection analysis guidelines.

AP Axial Coccyx Projection Analysis Guidelines
■ The coccyx is aligned with the (A) _____ and is at equal distances from the lateral walls of the (B) _____. ■ The first through (C) _____ coccygeal vertebrae are seen without foreshortening and without pubis symphysis superimposition.

100. How much can the transverse field be safely collimated and still include the required anatomic structures for an AP coccygeal projection?

_____

101. Why is the patient instructed to empty the bladder and colon before an AP sacral projection is taken? _____

_____

102. When a patient is rotated for an AP coccygeal projection, the coccyx rotates in the (A) _____ (opposite/same) direction as the pubis symphysis and is positioned next to the lateral pelvic wall situated (B) _____ (closer to/farther from) the IR.

103. How must the patient and CR be positioned for an AP coccygeal projection to demonstrate the coccyx without foreshortening?

_____

104. What is the curvature of the coccyx? _____

105. Accurate CR centering on an AP coccygeal projection is accomplished by positioning the CR to the (A) _____ plane at a level 2 inches (5 cm) superior to the (B) _____.

106. Which anatomic structures are included on an AP coccygeal projection with accurate positioning?

_____

For the following descriptions of AP coccygeal projections with poor positioning, state how the patient or CR would have been mispositioned for such a projection to be obtained.

107. The urinary bladder is dense and creating a shadow over the coccyx.

_____

108. The coccyx is not aligned with the pubis symphysis but is situated closer to the left lateral pelvic wall.

_____

109. The pubis symphysis is superimposed over the coccyx, and the second and third coccygeal vertebrae are foreshortened.

_____

For the following AP coccygeal projections with poor positioning, state which anatomic structures are misaligned and how the patient should be repositioned for an optimal projection to be obtained.

Figure 9-29

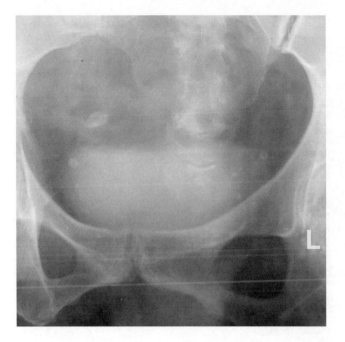

110. Figure 9-29: _____

_____

_____

Figure 9-30

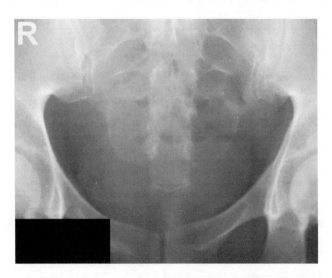

111. Figure 9-30: _____

_____

_____

Coccyx: Lateral Projection

112. Identify the labeled anatomy in Figure 9-31.

Figure 9-31

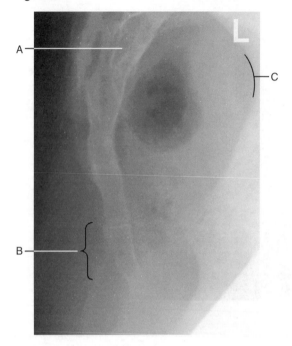

A. _____

B. _____

C. _____

113. Complete the statements below referring to lateral coccyx projection analysis guidelines.

Lateral Coccyx Projection Analysis Guidelines
■ The median sacral crest is in (A) _____, and the greater sciatic notches are superimposed.
■ The coccyx is seen without (B) _____.

114. How can rotation be detected on a rotated lateral coccygeal projection?

_____

115. How is the patient positioned to prevent foreshortening of the coccyx on a lateral coccygeal projection?

_____

_____

116. Accurate CR centering on a lateral coccygeal projection is accomplished by centering a perpendicular central ray approximately 3.5 inches (9 cm) (A) _____ and 2 inches (5 cm) (B) _____ to the elevated (C) _____.

117. How tightly can one safely collimate on a lateral coccygeal projection without fear of clipping any portion of the coccyx?

_____

118. Which anatomic structures are included on a lateral coccygeal projection with accurate positioning?

_____

For the following description of a lateral coccygeal projection with poor positioning, state how the patient would have been mispositioned for such a projection to be obtained.

119. The greater sciatic notches are demonstrated without superimposition, and the ischium is nearly superimposed over the third coccygeal segment.

_____

For the following lateral coccygeal projection with poor positioning, state which anatomic structures are misaligned and how the patient should be repositioned for an optimal projection to be obtained.

Figure 9-32

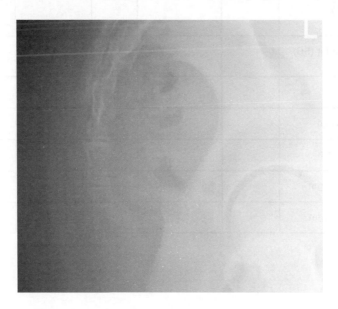

120. Figure 9-32: _____

_____

_____

10 Image Analysis of the Bony Thorax

STUDY QUESTIONS

1. Complete Figure 10-1.

Figure 10-1

Projection	kV	Grid	AEC	mAs	SID
PA oblique (RAO position), sternum					
PA sternoclavicular (SC) articulations					
PA oblique sternoclavicular (SC) articulations					
Lateral, sternum					
AP or PA, above diaphragm					
AP or PA, below diaphragm					
PA oblique, above diaphragm					
PA oblique, below diaphragm					

Sternum: PA Oblique Projection (RAO Position)

2. Identify the labeled anatomy in Figure 10-2.

Figure 10-2

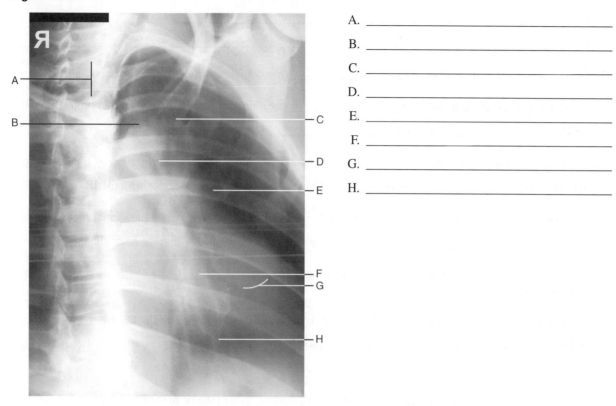

A. _____

B. _____

C. _____

D. _____

E. _____

F. _____

G. _____

H. _____

3. Complete the statements below referring to PA oblique sternum projection (RAO position) analysis guidelines.

PA Oblique Sternum Projection (RAO Position) Analysis Guidelines

■ The ribs and lung markings are (A) _____, and the posterior ribs and (B) _____ are magnified.

■ The manubrium, SC joints, sternal body, and xiphoid process are demonstrated within the heart shadow without

(C) _____ superimposition.

---

4. Why is a PA oblique (RAO) projection chosen over a PA oblique (LAO) projection when imaging the sternum?

_____

_____

5. Keeping the entire sternum within the heart shadow for the PA oblique projection provides a sternal projection that

demonstrates homogeneous (A) _____ across the entire sternum.

6. List four structures that overlie the sternum in a PA oblique sternal projection.

A. _____

B. _____

C. _____

D. _____

7. Using a short SID will result in (A) _____ (lower/higher) patient entrance skin dosage.

8. Using a long exposure time and (A) _____ breathing for the PA oblique sternal projection will blur the (B) _____ and (C) _____.

9. The sternum is rotated from beneath the thoracic vertebrae for a PA oblique sternal projection by rotating the patient until the (A) _____ plane is aligned (B) _____ degrees with the IR.

10. Any portion of the sternum that is positioned outside the heart shadow on a PA oblique sternal projection demonstrates (A) _____ (more/less) brightness than that positioned within the heart shadow.

11. On a PA oblique sternal projection with accurate positioning, the (A) _____ is centered within the collimated field.

12. Proper centering for a PA oblique sternal projection is accomplished by centering the CR (A) _____ inch(es) to the left of the (B) _____ and placing the top of the IR approximately 1.5 inches superior to the (C) _____.

13. Because the long axis of the sternum does not align with the long axis of the IR in the PA oblique sternal projection, transverse collimation should be limited to the (A) _____ and (B) _____.

For the following description of a PA oblique sternal projection with poor positioning, state how the patient would have been mispositioned for such a projection to be obtained.

14. The right sternoclavicular (SC) joint and right side of the manubrium are superimposed by the thoracic vertebrae.

_____

_____

For the following PA oblique sternal projections with poor positioning, state which anatomic structures are misaligned and how the patient should be repositioned for an optimal projection to be obtained.

Figure 10-3

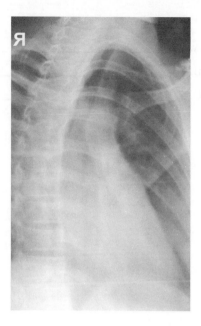

15. Figure 10-3: _____

_____

_____

_____

Figure 10-4

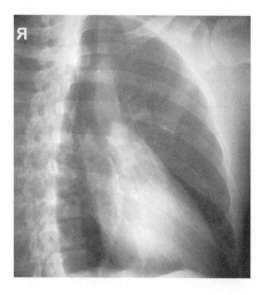

16. Figure 10-4: _____

_____

_____

_____

Sternum: Lateral Projection

17. Identify the labeled anatomy in Figure 10-5.

Figure 10-5

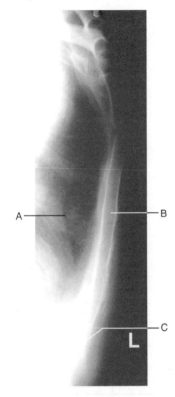

A. _____

B. _____

C. _____

18. Identify the labeled anatomy in Figure 10-6.

Figure 10-6

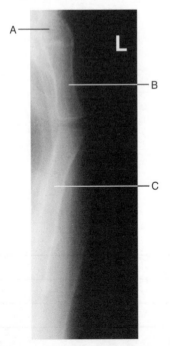

A. _____

B. _____

C. _____

19. Complete the statements below referring to lateral sternum projection analysis guidelines.

Lateral Sternum Projection Analysis Guidelines

- The manubrium, sternal body, and xiphoid process are in (A) _____, and the anterior ribs are not superimposed over the sternum.

- No superimposition of (B) _____ soft tissue over the sternum is present.

- The (C) _____ is at the center of the exposure field.

---

20. Why is it often difficult to demonstrate the superior and inferior sternum simultaneously on a lateral sternal projection?

_____

_____

21. List three methods of controlling the amount of scatter radiation that reaches the IR on a lateral sternal projection.

A. _____

B. _____

C. _____

22. How is rotation avoided when positioning the patient for a lateral sternal projection?

_____

23. Describe how one can determine on a lateral sternal projection with poor positioning that the patient's right thorax is rotated anteriorly.

_____

24. Deep suspended respiration draws the sternum away from the _____.

25. How is the patient positioned to prevent humeral soft tissue from superimposing the sternum?

_____

26. Accurate CR centering on a lateral sternal projection is accomplished by placing the top edge of the IR

(A) _____ inch(es) above the (B) _____ and aligning the receptor's long axis and a(n)

(C) _____ CR to the midsternum.

27. Why is a 72-inch (180-cm) SID used for a lateral sternum projection?

_____

_____

28. Which anatomic structures are included on a lateral sternal projection with accurate positioning?

_____

429

For the following descriptions of lateral sternal projections with poor positioning, state how the patient would have been mispositioned for such a projection to be obtained.

29. The anterior ribs are demonstrated without superimposition, the sternum is not in profile, and the superior heart shadow extends beyond the sternum and into the anteriorly situated lung.

_____

30. The anterior ribs are demonstrated without superimposition, the sternum is not in profile, and the superior heart shadow does not extend beyond the sternum.

_____

For the following lateral sternal projection with poor positioning, state which anatomic structures are misaligned and how the patient should be repositioned for an optimal projection to be obtained.

Figure 10-7

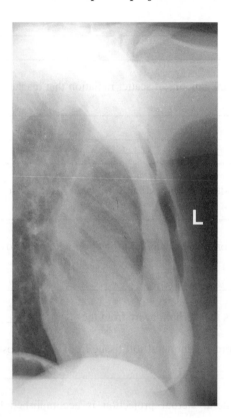

31. Figure 10-7: _____

_____

_____

_____

_____

Sternoclavicular (SC) Articulations: PA Projection

32. Complete the statements below referring to PA SC articulations projection analysis guidelines.

SC Articulations PA Projection Analysis Guidelines

- Distances from the vertebral column to the (A) _____ clavicular ends are (B) _____.
- The (C) _____ is not in the exposure field.
- Clavicles are positioned on the same (D) _____ plane.

---

33. Accurate CR centering on a PA SC articulations projection is accomplished by centering a (A) _____ CR at a level (B) _____ inches inferior to the (C) _____.

34. What anatomic structures are included on a PA SC articulations projection? _____

_____.

For the following PA SC articulations projection with poor positioning, state which anatomic structures are mis-aligned and how the patient should be repositioned for an optimal projection to be obtained.

Figure 10-8

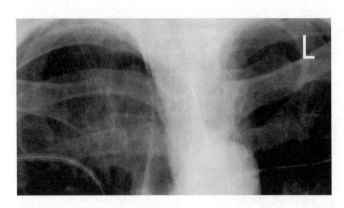

35. Figure 10-8:_____

Sternoclavicular (SC) Articulations: PA Oblique Projection

36. Complete the statements below referring to PA oblique SC articulations projection analysis guidelines.

SC Articulations PA Oblique Projection Analysis Guidelines

- SC articulation is demonstrated next to the (A) _____ and without spinal (B) _____.
- Clavicles are positioned on the (C) _____ horizontal plane.
- SC articulation of (D) _____ is in the center of the exposure field.

431

37. Accurate CR centering on a PA oblique SC articulations projection is obtained by positioning the CR at a level 3 inches (7.5 cm) (A) _____ to the vertebral prominins and (B) _____inches lateral to the (C) _____ plane.

38. What anatomic structures are included on a PA oblique SC articulations projection?

_____.

For the following PA SC articulations projection with poor positioning, state which anatomic structures are misaligned and how the patient should be repositioned for an optimal projection to be obtained.

Figure 10-9

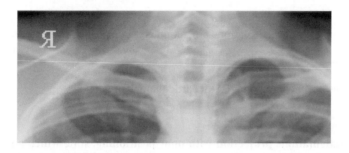

39. Figure 10-9: _____

Ribs: AP or PA Projection

40. Identify the labeled anatomy in Figure 10-10.

Figure 10-10

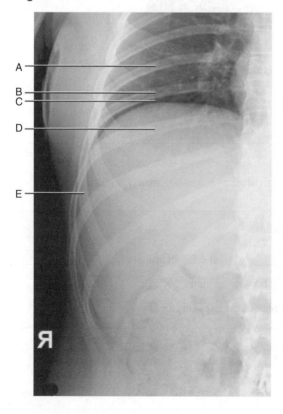

A. _____

B. _____

C. _____

D. _____

E. _____

41. Complete the statements below referring to AP/PA rib projection analysis guidelines.

> **AP or PA Rib Projection Analysis Guidelines**
>
> - Thoracic vertebrae–rib head articulations are demonstrated, the medial clavicular end is adjacent to the lateral edge of the (A) _____, and the distances from the (B) _____ to the pedicles on each side, when seen, are equal.
> - Above the diaphragm: Scapulae are outside the lung field, and (C) _____ posterior ribs are seen above the diaphragm.
> - Below the diaphragm: The (D) _____ through 12th posterior ribs are included within the exposure.

42. Why do some facilities require the technologist to tape a rib marker (lead "BB") on the patient's skin near the area where the ribs are tender?

_____

_____

43. What patient respiration is used when imaging ribs located above the diaphragm?

A. _____

_____

What patient respiration is used when imaging ribs located below the diaphragm?

B. _____

_____

44. What soft tissue structures are evaluated for associated injury on the following rib projections?

A. Upper ribs: _____

_____

B. Lower ribs: _____

_____

45. If the patient complains of anterior rib pain, what projection of the ribs should be taken?

A. (AP/PA) _____

When the patient indicates posterior rib pain, what projection of the ribs should be taken?

B. (AP/PA) _____

If the opposite is taken for these two situations, what difference would result?

C. _____

46. How is spinal scoliosis identified on PA and AP rib projections?

_____

_____

47. Accurate CR centering on an above-diaphragm AP rib projection is accomplished by centering the CR halfway between the (A) _____ and affected lateral rib surface, at a level halfway between the (B) _____ and (C) _____. This centering is accomplished on a PA projection by placing the CR halfway between the (D) _____ and affected lateral rib surface at the level of the (E) _____.

48. Which anatomic structures are included on an above-diaphragm AP or PA rib projection with accurate positioning?

    _____

    _____

49. Accurate CR centering on a below-diaphragm AP or PA rib projection is accomplished by placing the lower border of the IR at the (A) _____, centering a perpendicular CR to the IR, and moving the patient side to side until the longitudinal collimator light line is aligned halfway between the (B) _____ and affected lateral rib surface.

50. Which anatomic structures are included on an AP or PA below-diaphragm rib projection with accurate positioning?

    _____

    _____

For the following descriptions of AP or PA rib projections with poor positioning, state how the patient would have been mispositioned for such a projection to be obtained.

51. The medial clavicular end is situated away from the lateral edge of the vertebral column on an AP projection taken because of left rib pain.

    _____

    _____

52. The left scapula is superimposed over the upper lateral rib field on a PA projection.

    _____

    _____

53. The 10th through 12th posterior ribs are demonstrated below the diaphragm on a below-diaphragm projection.

    _____

    _____

For the following AP or PA rib projections with poor positioning, state which anatomic structures are misaligned and how the patient should be repositioned for an optimal projection to be obtained.

Figure 10-11

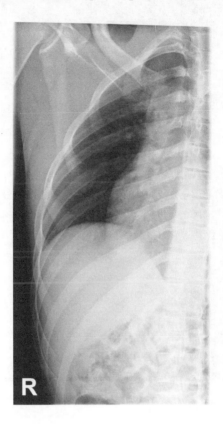

54. Figure 10-11, AP projection, above-diaphragm ribs:

_____

_____

_____

_____

Figure 10-12

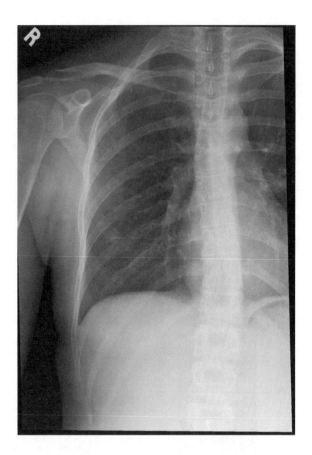

55. Figure 10-12, AP projection, above-diaphragm ribs:

_____

_____

Figure 10-13

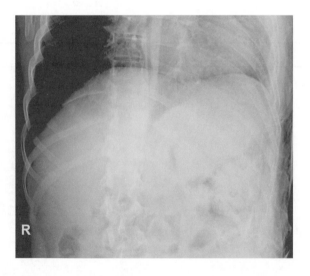

56. Figure 10-13, AP projection, below-diaphragm ribs:

_____

_____

_____

Ribs: AP Oblique Projection (RPO and LPO Positions)

57. Identify the labeled anatomy in Figure 10-14.

Figure 10-14

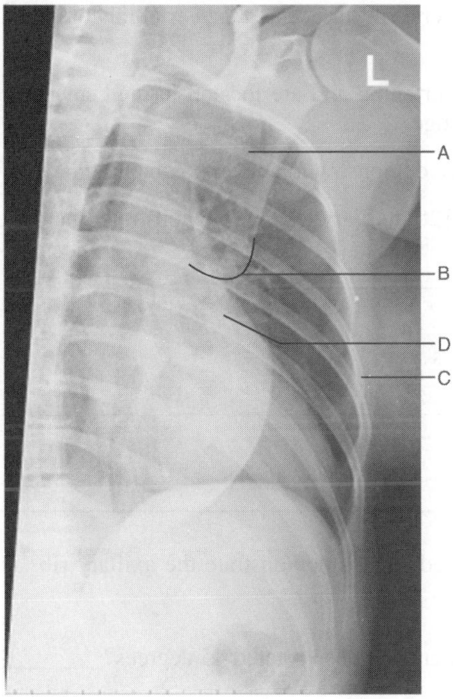

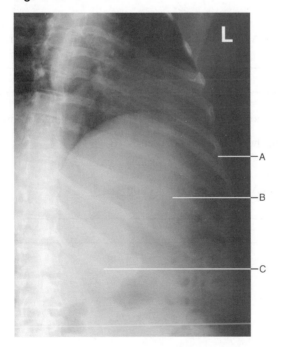

A. _____

B. _____

C. _____

D. _____

58. Identify the labeled anatomy in Figure 10-15.

Figure 10-15

A. _____

B. _____

C. _____

59. Complete the statements below referring to AP oblique ribs projection analysis guidelines.

AP Oblique Rib Projection Analysis Guidelines

- The (A) _____ is located halfway between the lateral rib surface and the vertebral column, and the axillary ribs are free of superimposition.

- The (B) _____ are demonstrated without foreshortening and are located in the center of the collimated field, and the anterior ribs are located at the lateral edge.

- Above the diaphragm: (C) _____ axillary ribs are demonstrated above the diaphragm.

- Below the diaphragm: The (D) _____ through 12th axillary ribs are demonstrated below the diaphragm.

---

60. What degree of patient rotation is used for AP oblique rib projections?

A. _____

Which body plane is used to align this angle?

B. _____

61. State whether the patient is rotated toward or away from the affected side to demonstrate the axillary ribs in the AP oblique projection. _____

62. How can one determine from an AP oblique rib projection if the patient has been rotated 45 degrees? _____

_____

63. Accurate CR centering on an above-diaphragm AP oblique rib projection is accomplished by centering a(n)

(A) _____ CR halfway between the midsagittal plane and (B) _____ at a level

halfway between the (C) _____ and (D) _____.

64. Which anatomic structures are included on an above-diaphragm AP oblique rib projection with accurate positioning?

_____

_____

65. Accurate CR centering on a below-diaphragm AP oblique rib projection is accomplished by positioning the lower

IR border at the patient's (A) _____ and centering the CR halfway between the (B) _____ and affected lateral rib surface.

66. Which anatomic structures are included on a below-diaphragm AP oblique rib projection?

_____

_____

For the following descriptions of AP oblique rib projections with poor positioning, state how the patient would have been mispositioned for such a projection to be obtained.

67. The axillary ribs demonstrate increased foreshortening, and the sternum is rotated toward the patient's left side on a projection taken for right side rib pain.

_____

_____

68. The sternal body is demonstrated adjacent to the vertebral column.

_____

_____

69. An above-diaphragm AP oblique rib projection demonstrates the first through seventh posterior ribs above the diaphragm.

_____

_____

For the following AP and PA oblique rib projections with poor positioning, state which anatomic structures are misaligned and how the patient should be repositioned for an optimal projection to be obtained.

Figure 10-16

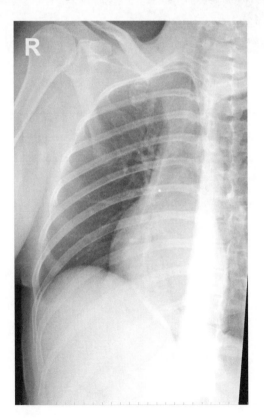

70. Figure 10-16, AP oblique projection:

_____

_____

Figure 10-17

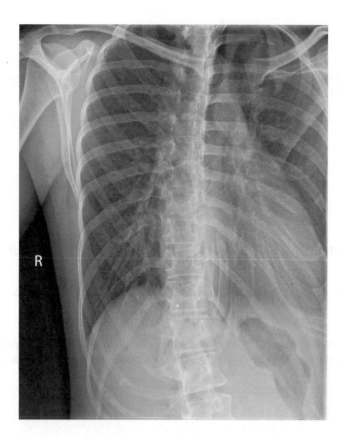

71. Figure 10-17, below-diaphragm AP oblique projection:

_____

_____

_____

11 Image Analysis of the Cranium

STUDY QUESTIONS

1. Complete Figure 11-1.

Figure 11-1

Cranium, Facial Bones, and Paranasal Sinus Technical Data						
Projection	Structure	kV	Grid	AEC	mAs	SID
AP or PA						
PA axial (Caldwell method)						
AP axial (Towne method)						
Lateral						
Submentovertex (Schueller method)						
Pariet oacanthial (Waters method)						

2. State the cranial positioning lines indicated in Figure 11-2.

Figure 11-2

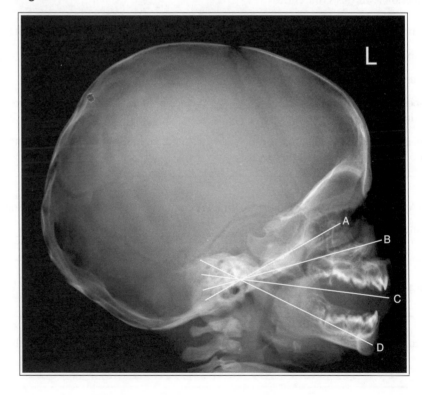

A. _____

B. _____

C. _____

D. _____

Cranium and Mandible: PA or AP Projection

3. Identify the labeled anatomy in Figure 11-3.

Figure 11-3

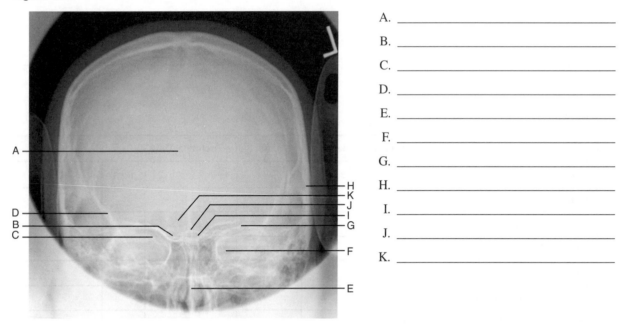

A. _____

B. _____

C. _____

D. _____

E. _____

F. _____

G. _____

H. _____

I. _____

J. _____

K. _____

4. Complete the statements below referring to PA cranial and mandibular projection analysis guidelines.

PA Cranium and Mandible Projection Analysis Guidelines

■ The distances from the lateral margin of orbits to the lateral cranial (A) _____ and from the mandibular (B) _____ to the lateral cervical vertebrae on both sides are equal.

■ The anterior clinoids and dorsum sellae are seen superior to the (C) _____.

■ The petrous ridges are superimposed over the (D) _____, and the internal acoustic meatus are visualized horizontally through the center of the orbits.

■ The (E) _____ is aligned with the long axis of the exposure field, and the supraorbital margins and the TMJs are demonstrated on the same horizontal plane.

---

5. The midsagittal plane is positioned (A) _____ to the IR for a PA cranial projection to prevent rotation.

How is this positioning best accomplished? (B) _____

_____

6. How is cranial rotation identified on a rotated PA skull projection?

_____

7. How is the patient's head position adjusted to prevent rotation on an AP skull projection taken in a patient with a suspected cervical injury?

_____

8. PA and AP skull projections demonstrate different magnified anatomic structures. Which of these projections demonstrates the greater orbital magnification?

A. _____

Which projection demonstrates the greater parietal bone magnification?

B. _____

9. Which cranial positioning line is used to obtain an accurate PA projection? (A) _____ How is this

line positioned with respect to the IR? (B) _____

10. If the patient is unable to accurately position the line indicated in the previous question to the IR for a PA cranial projection, how is the CR adjusted to compensate?

_____

11. When the patient's chin is tucked for a PA cranial projection, in which direction will the supraorbital margins move

with respect to the petrous ridges? _____ (inferiorly/superiorly)

12. If the patient is unable to adjust the degree of chin elevation for an AP trauma cranial projection, how is the CR used to compensate?

_____

13. A PA skull projection with poor positioning demonstrates approximately 1 inch (2.5 cm) of space between the petrous ridges and supraorbital margins. The ridges are inferior. Where are the dorsum sellae and anterior clinoids

demonstrated with respect to the ethmoid sinuses on this projection? _____

14. On a trauma AP cranial projection with poor positioning, the petrous ridges are demonstrated superior to the supraorbital margins. The distance between them is approximately 0.5 inch (1.25 cm). Will there be an increase or decrease in the amount of dorsum sella and anterior clinoid superimposition above the ethmoid sinuses on this projection?

_____

15. Which anatomic structure is aligned with the long axis on the projection if the patient's midsagittal plane is accurately aligned with the collimated field on a PA or AP cranial projection?

_____

16. On a PA or AP cranial projection with accurate positioning, the (A) _____ is centered within the

collimated field. This centering is obtained when the CR is centered to the (B) _____.

17. Which anatomic structures are included on a PA or AP cranial projection with accurate positioning?

_____

18. On a PA or AP mandible projection with accurate positioning, the (A) _____ is centered within the

exposure field. This centering is obtained when the CR is centered to (B) _____.

19. Which anatomic structures are included on a PA or AP mandibular projection with accurate positioning?

_____

For the following descriptions of PA cranial projections with poor positioning, state how the patient or CR would have been mispositioned for such an image to be obtained.

20. The distance from the lateral orbital margins to the lateral cranial cortex on the left side is greater than on the right side.

_____

21. The petrous ridges are demonstrated inferior to the supraorbital margins, and the dorsum sellae and anterior clinoids are superimposed over the ethmoid sinuses. How was the patient mispositioned?

    A. _____

    If this were a trauma AP projection, how would the CR have been mispositioned?

    B. _____

22. The petrous ridges are demonstrated superior to the supraorbital margins. How was the patient mispositioned?

    A. _____

    If this were a trauma AP projection, how would the CR have been mispositioned?

    B. _____

For the following PA cranial projections with poor positioning, state which anatomic structures are misaligned and how the patient should be repositioned for an optimal image to be obtained.

Figure 11-4

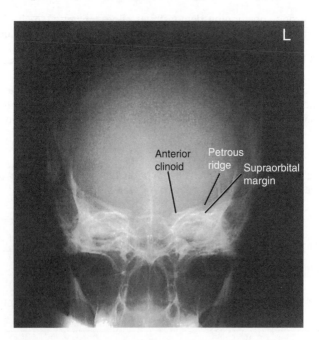

23. Figure 11-4, PA projection: _____

_____

_____

_____

444

Figure 11-5

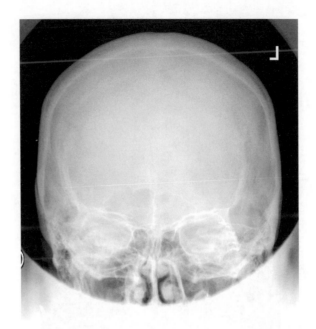

24. Figure 11-5, PA projection: _____

_____

_____

_____

Figure 11-6

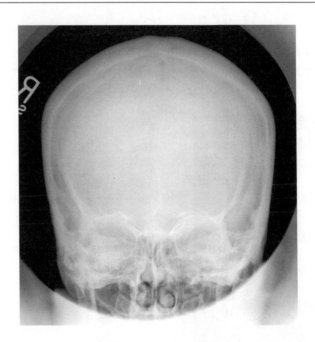

25. Figure 11-6, PA projection: _____

_____

_____

_____

Chapter **11 Image Analysis of the Cranium**

Figure 11-7

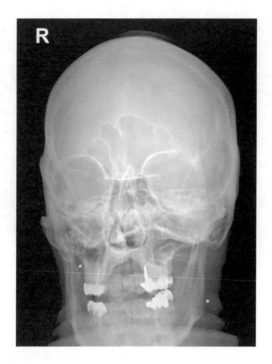

26. Figure 11-7, AP projection, trauma: _____

_____

_____

_____

Cranium, Facial Bones, and Sinuses: PA Axial Projection (Caldwell Method)

27. Identify the labeled anatomy in Figure 11-8.

Figure 11-8

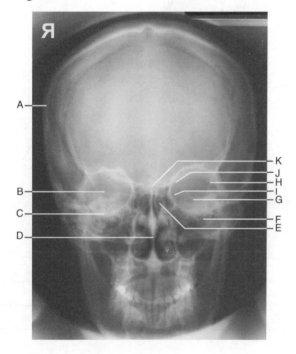

A. _____

B. _____

C. _____

D. _____

E. _____

F. _____

G. _____

H. _____

I. _____

J. _____

K. _____

28. Complete the statements below referring to PA axial cranial, facial bones, and sinuses projection analysis guidelines.

> **PA Axial Cranium, Facial Bones, and Sinuses Projection Analysis Guidelines**
>
> - The distances from the lateral orbital margins to the (A) _____ on both sides are equal.
> - The petrous ridges are demonstrated horizontally through the lower third of the (B) _____, the petrous pyramids are superimposed over the (C) _____, and the superior orbital fissures are seen within the orbits.
> - The (D) _____ is aligned with the long axis of the exposure field, and the supraorbital margins are demonstrated on the same horizontal plane.

29. Which plane is positioned perpendicular to the IR for a PA axial projection?

    _____

30. When rotation is present on a PA axial projection, the patient's face is rotated (A) _____ (toward/away from) the side of the cranium that demonstrates the greater distance. On an AP axial projection, the patient's face is rotated (B) _____ (toward/away from) the side of the cranium that demonstrates the greater distance.

31. What are the degree and direction of the CR angulation used on a PA axial projection of the cranium?

    _____

32. What are the degree and direction of the CR angulation used on an AP axial projection of the cranium when the patient is capable of adequately positioning the head?

    _____

33. Accurate positioning for a PA or AP axial cranial projection is obtained when the _____ line is aligned perpendicular to the IR.

34. How is the CR angulation determined for a PA axial cranial projection of a patient who is unable to accurately position the head? _____

    _____

35. What is the CR angulation for a PA axial projection of the cranium for a patient who can tuck the chin only enough to place the OML at a 10-degree cephalad angle with the IR?

    _____

36. What is the CR angulation for an AP axial projection of the cranium for a patient who can tuck the chin only enough to place the OML at a 5-degree caudal angle with the IR?

    _____

37. On a PA and AP axial projection with accurate positioning, the (A) _____ are centered within the exposure field. This is accomplished by centering the CR to (B) _____.

38. Which anatomic structures are included on a PA or AP axial projection of the cranium with accurate positioning?

A. _____

On a projection of facial bones or sinuses?

B. _____

For the following descriptions of PA axial cranial projections with poor positioning, state how the patient or CR would have been mispositioned for such an image to be obtained.

39. The distance from the lateral orbital margin to the lateral cranial cortex on the left side is greater than that on the right side. How was the patient mispositioned for this image?

_____

40. The petrous ridges are demonstrated inferior to the inferior orbital margins. How was the patient mispositioned for such a projection to be obtained if the CR was accurately angled?

A. _____

How was the CR mispositioned for such a projection to be obtained if the patient was accurately positioned?

B. _____

41. The petrous ridges and pyramids are superior to the supraorbital margins, and the internal auditory canals are distorted. How was the patient mispositioned for such a projection to be obtained if the CR was accurately angled?

A. _____

How was the CR mispositioned for such a projection to be obtained if the patient was accurately positioned?

B. _____

For the following PA axial cranial projections with poor positioning, state which anatomic structures are misaligned and how the patient should be repositioned for an optimal image to be obtained.

Figure 11-9

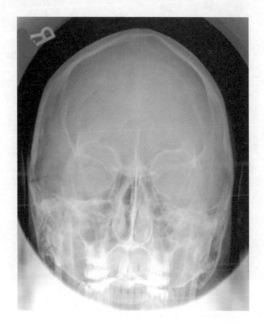

42. Figure 11-9, PA axial projection: _____

_____

_____

_____

Figure 11-10

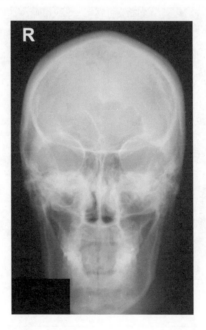

43. Figure 11-10, AP axial projection, trauma: _____

_____

_____

_____

Chapter **11 Image Analysis of the Cranium**

Figure 11-11

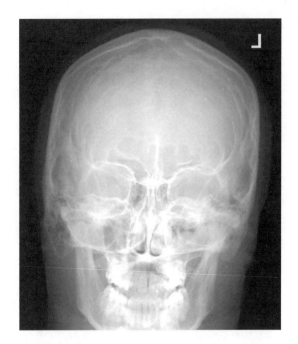

44. Figure 11-11, PA axial projection: _____

_____

_____

_____

Figure 11-12

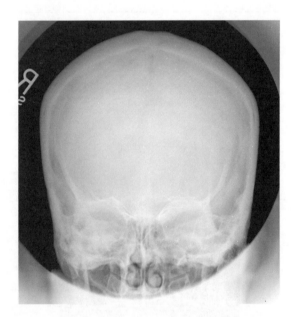

45. Figure 11-12, PA axial projection: _____

_____

_____

_____

Cranium and Mandible: AP Axial Projection (Towne Method)

46. Identify the labeled anatomy in Figure 11-13.

Figure 11-13

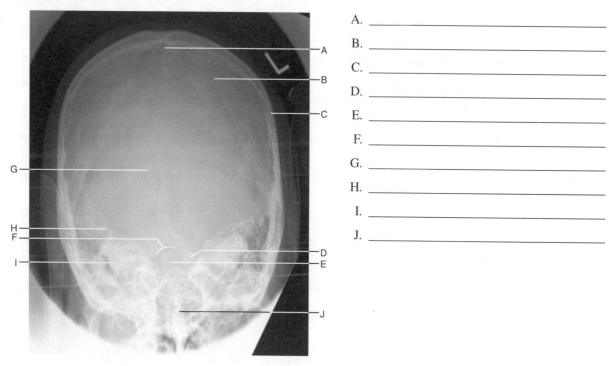

A. _____

B. _____

C. _____

D. _____

E. _____

F. _____

G. _____

H. _____

I. _____

J. _____

47. Identify the labeled anatomy in Figure 11-14.

Figure 11-14

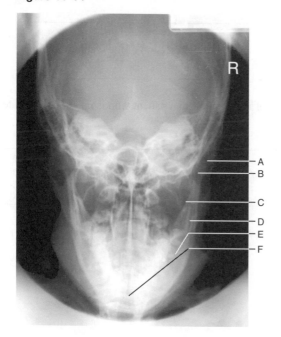

A. _____

B. _____

C. _____

D. _____

E. _____

F. _____

48. Complete the statements below referring to AP axial cranial and mandibular projection analysis guidelines.

> **AP Axial Cranium and Mandible Projection Analysis Guidelines**
>
> - The distances from the posterior clinoid process to the lateral borders of the (A) _____ on both sides and the mandibular necks to the lateral cervical vertebrae on both sides are equal, the petrous ridges are symmetrical, and the dorsum sellae is centered within the (B) _____.
> - Cranium: The dorsum sellae and (C) _____ are seen within the foramen magnum without foreshortening or superimposition of the atlas's posterior arch.
> - Mandible: The dorsum sellae and posterior clinoids are at the level of the (D) _____ foramen magnum, and the mandibular condyles and fossae are clearly demonstrated, with minimal mastoid superimposition.
> - The (E) _____ and nasal septum are aligned with the long axis of the exposure field.

49. The (A) _____ plane is positioned (B) _____ to the IR to prevent rotation on an AP axial projection.

50. When rotation is present on an AP axial projection, the side demonstrating less distance between the posterior clinoid process and the lateral border of the foramen magnum is the side (A) _____ (toward/away from) which the patient's face is rotated.

51. When the correct CR angulation and head position are used on an AP axial projection, the (A) _____ and posterior clinoids are demonstrated within the (B) _____.

52. What are the degree and direction of the CR angulation used on an AP axial projection of the cranium and mandible?

_____

53. Which cranial positioning line is aligned perpendicular to the IR for an AP axial projection of the cranium?

_____

54. How is the CR angulation determined for an AP axial projection of the cranium in a patient who is unable to accurately position the head?

_____

55. Which anatomic structures are included on an AP axial projection of the cranium with accurate positioning?

_____

For the following descriptions of AP axial projections of the cranium with inaccurate positioning, state how the patient or CR would have been mispositioned for such an image to be obtained.

56. The distance from the posterior clinoid process to the lateral foramen magnum on the patient's left side is less than that on the patient's right side.

_____

57. The dorsum sellae and anterior clinoids are demonstrated superior to the foramen magnum. How would the patient have been mispositioned for such a projection to be obtained if the CR was accurately angled?

A. _____

How would the CR have been mispositioned for such a projection to be obtained if the patient was accurately positioned?

B. _____

58. The dorsum sella is foreshortened and superimposed over the atlas's posterior arch. How would the patient have been mispositioned for such a projection to be obtained if the CR was accurately angled?

A. _____

How would the CR have been mispositioned for such a projection to be obtained if the patient was accurately positioned?

B. _____

For the following AP axial projections of the cranium and mandible with poor positioning, state which anatomic structures are misaligned and how the patient should be repositioned for an optimal image to be obtained.

Figure 11-15

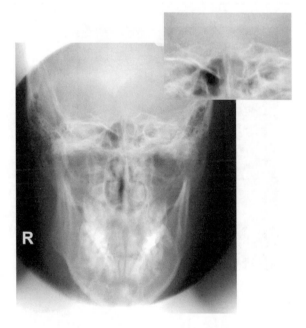

59. Figure 11-15: _____

_____

_____

_____

Figure 11-16

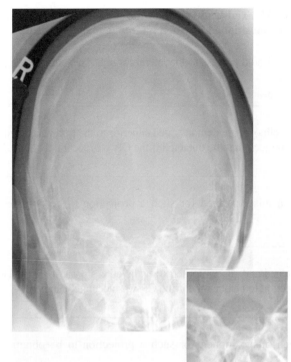

60. Figure 11-16: _____

_____

_____

_____

Figure 11-17

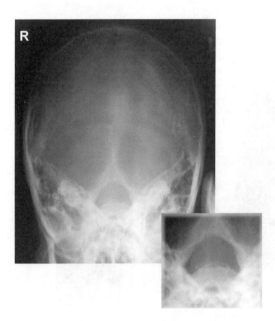

61. Figure 11-17: _____

_____

_____

Cranium, Facial Bones, Nasal Bones, and Sinuses: Lateral Projection

62. Identify the labeled anatomy in Figure 11-18.

Figure 11-18

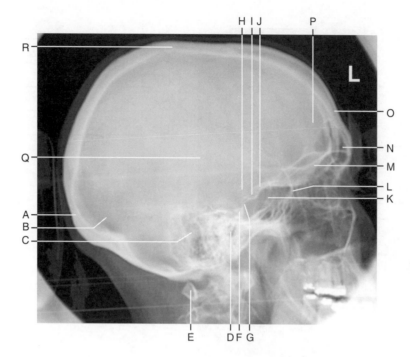

A. _____   J. _____

B. _____   K. _____

C. _____   L. _____

D. _____   M. _____

E. _____   N. _____

F. _____   O. _____

G. _____   P. _____

H. _____   Q. _____

I. _____   R. _____

63. Identify the labeled anatomy in Figure 11-19.

Figure 11-19

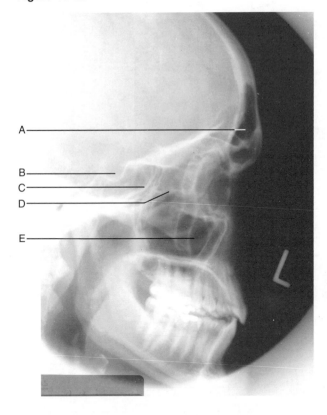

A. _____

B. _____

C. _____

D. _____

E. _____

64. Identify the labeled anatomy in Figure 11-20.

Figure 11-20

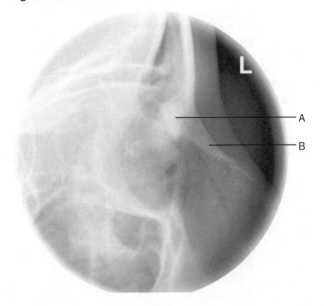

A. _____

B. _____

65. Complete the statements below referring to lateral cranium, facial and nasal bones, and sinuses projection analysis guidelines.

Lateral Cranium, Facial and Nasal Bones, and Sinuses Projection Analysis Guidelines

- When visualized, the sella turcica is seen in (A) _____. Orbital roofs, mandibular rami, greater wings of the sphenoid, external acoustic canals, zygomatic bones, and cranial cortices are

  (B) _____.

- Cranium: The posteroinferior occipital bones and (C) _____ of the atlas are free of superimposition.

---

66. Which sinuses are demonstrated on a lateral projection of the sinuses?

_____

67. Why is it best to take a lateral sinus projection with the patient in an upright position?

_____

68. Which plane is used to position the patient to prevent rotation and tilting on a lateral cranial projection?

A. _____

How is it aligned with the IR?

B. _____

How does this positioning align the interpupillary (IP) line with the IR?

C. _____

69. How is the patient or IR positioned to include the occipital bone for a lateral cranial projection of a recumbent patient without cervical trauma?

A. _____

Of a recumbent patient with cervical trauma?

B. _____

70. How can cranial tilting be distinguished from rotation on a lateral cranial projection?

_____

_____

71. How is the patient positioned to ensure that the posteroinferior occipital bone and posterior arch of the atlas are free of superimposition?

_____

72. On a lateral cranial projection with accurate positioning, the CR is centered 2 inches (5 cm) (A) _____ to the

(B) _____.

73. Which anatomic structures are included on a lateral cranial projection with accurate positioning?

_____

74. On a lateral sinus projection with accurate positioning, the (A) _____ and greater wings of the sphenoid are centered within the exposure field. This is accomplished by centering the CR halfway between the

(B) _____ and (C) _____.

75. Which anatomic structures are included on a lateral sinus projection with accurate positioning?

_____

76. On a lateral nasal projection with accurate positioning, the (A) _____ are centered within the exposure field. This is accomplished by centering the CR 0.5 inch (1.25 cm) (B) _____ to the nasion.

77. Which anatomic structures are included on a lateral nasal bone projection with accurate positioning?

_____

For the following descriptions of lateral cranial projections with poor positioning, state how the patient would have been mispositioned for such an image to be obtained.

78. The greater wings of the sphenoid and the anterior cranial cortices are demonstrated without superimposition. One of each corresponding structure is demonstrated anterior to the other.

_____

79. The orbital roofs, external auditory meatus, and inferior cranial cortices are demonstrated without superimposition. One of each corresponding structure is demonstrated superior to the other, and the foramen is not visualized.

_____

For the following lateral cranial projections with poor positioning, state which anatomic structures are misaligned and how the patient should be repositioned for an optimal image to be obtained.

Figure 11-21

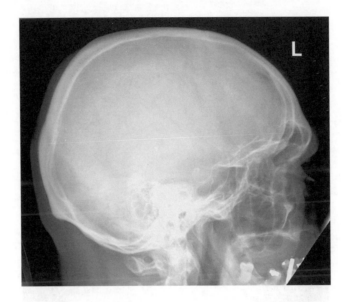

80. Figure 11-21: _____

_____

_____

_____

Figure 11-22

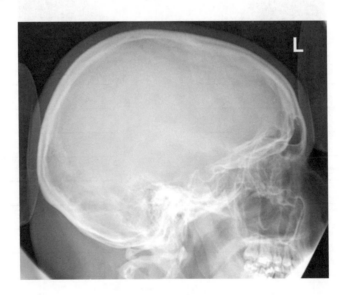

81. Figure 11-22: _____

_____

_____

_____

Cranium, Mandible, and Sinuses: Submentovertex (SMV) Projection (Schueller Method)

82. Identify the labeled anatomy in Figure 11-23.

Figure 11-23

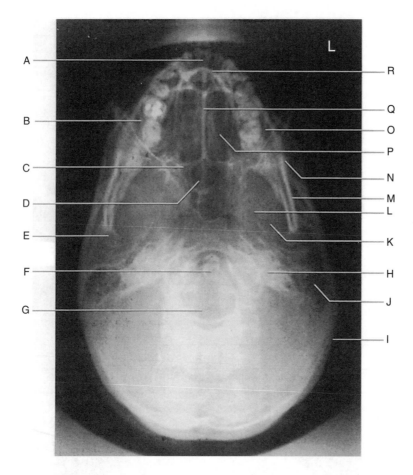

A. _____   J. _____

B. _____   K. _____

C. _____   L. _____

D. _____   M. _____

E. _____   N. _____

F. _____   O. _____

G. _____   P. _____

H. _____   Q. _____

I. _____   R. _____

83. Complete the statements below referring to SMV cranial, mandibular, and sinuses projection analysis guidelines.

> **Submentovertex (SMV) Cranium, Mandible, and Sinuses Projection Analysis Guidelines**
>
> - The mandibular mentum and nasal fossae are demonstrated just anterior to the (A) _____.
> - The distances from the mandibular ramus and body to the (B) _____ on both sides are equal.
> - The vomer, bony nasal septum, and (C) _____ are aligned with the long axis of the exposure field.

84. Accurate mandibular mentum and nasal fossae positioning on a SMV cranial projection is obtained when the

    (A) _____ cranial positioning line is aligned (B) _____ with the IR.

85. How is the positioning setup adjusted for a SMV cranial projection in a patient who is unable to extend the neck as far as needed?

    _____

86. How is cranial tilting identified on a tilted SMV cranial projection?

    A. _____

    How is the patient positioned to prevent tilting on a SMV cranial projection?

    B. _____

87. On a SMV cranial projection with accurate positioning, the (A) _____ is centered within the exposure

    field. This is accomplished when the CR is centered to the (B) _____ plane at a level

    (C) _____ inch(es) anterior to the level of the (D) _____.

88. Which anatomic structures are included on a SMV cranial projection with accurate positioning?

    _____

89. On a SMV sinus and mandible image with accurate positioning, the (A) _____ are centered within the

    collimated field. This is accomplished by centering the CR to the (B) _____ plane at a level

    (C) _____ inch(es) inferior to the (D) _____.

90. Which anatomic structures are included on a SMV sinus and mandible projection with accurate positioning?

    _____

For the following descriptions of SMV cranial projections with poor positioning, state how the patient or CR would have been mispositioned for such an image to be obtained.

91. The mandibular mentum is demonstrated too far anterior to the ethmoid sinuses.

    _____

92. The mandibular mentum is demonstrated posterior to the ethmoid sinuses. How would the patient have been mispositioned?

A. _____

How would the CR have been mispositioned?

B. _____

93. The distance from the left mandibular ramus and body to its corresponding lateral cranial cortex is greater than the distance from the right mandibular ramus and body to its corresponding lateral cranial cortex.

_____

For the following SMV cranial, facial bone, and sinus projections with poor positioning, state which anatomic structures are misaligned and how the patient should be repositioned for an optimal image to be obtained.

Figure 11-24

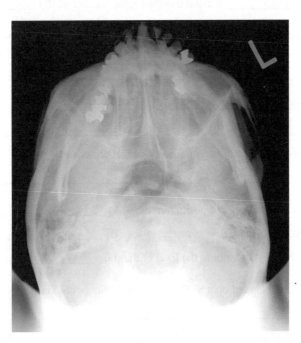

94. Figure 11-24: _____

_____

_____

_____

Figure 11-25

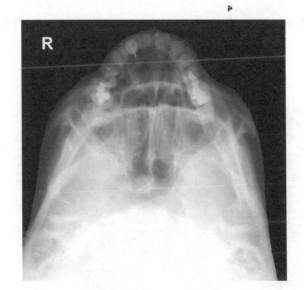

95. Figure 11-25: _____
_____
_____
_____
_____
_____

Figure 11-26

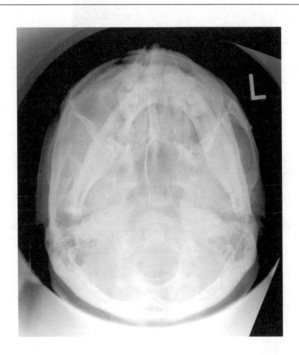

96. Figure 11-26: _____
_____
_____
_____

463

Facial Bones and Sinuses: Parietoacanthial and Acanthioparietal Projection (Waters and Open-Mouth Waters Methods)

97. Identify the labeled anatomy in Figure 11-27.

Figure 11-27

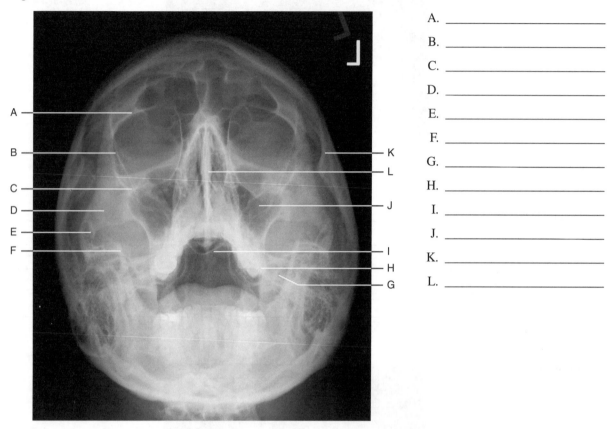

A. _____

B. _____

C. _____

D. _____

E. _____

F. _____

G. _____

H. _____

I. _____

J. _____

K. _____

L. _____

98. Complete the statements below referring to parietoacanthial and acanthioparietal facial bones and sinuses projection analysis guidelines.

Parietoacanthial and Acanthioparietal Facial Bones and Sinuses Projection Analysis Guidelines
■ The distances from the (A) _____ to the lateral cranial cortex on both sides are equal.
■ The petrous ridges are demonstrated (B) _____ to the maxillary sinuses and extend (C) _____ from the posterior maxillary alveolar process.
■ The bony nasal septum is aligned with the long axis of the exposure field, and the (D) _____ are demonstrated on the same horizontal plane.

99. Which sinuses are demonstrated on an open-mouth parietoacanthial projection that are not demonstrated on a closed-mouth parietoacanthial projection? _____

100. When rotation is present on a parietoacanthial projection, the patient's face is rotated (A) _____ (toward/away from) the side of the cranium that demonstrates the greatest distance. If an acanthioparietal projection is taken, the patient's face is rotated (B) _____ (toward/away from) the side of the cranium that demonstrates the greatest distance.

101. How is the patient positioned to accurately demonstrate the petrous ridges inferior to the maxillary sinuses on a parieto-acanthial projection? _____

102. On a parietoacanthial projection with accurate positioning, the (A) _____ is centered within the exposure field. This is accomplished by centering the CR to the (B) _____ .

103. Which anatomic structures are included on a parietoacanthial projection with accurate positioning?

_____

_____

For the following descriptions of parietoacanthial cranial projections with poor positioning, state how the patient would have been mispositioned for such a projection to be obtained.

104. The distances from the lateral orbital margin to the lateral cranial cortex on the left side of the patient are greater than the distances on the right side.

_____

_____

105. The petrous ridges are demonstrated within the maxillary sinuses and superior to the posterior maxillary alveolar process.

_____

_____

106. The petrous ridges are inferior to the maxillary sinuses and posterior maxillary alveolar process.

_____

_____

For the following parietoacanthial projections with poor positioning, state which anatomic structures are misaligned and how the patient should be repositioned for an optimal image to be obtained.

Figure 11-28

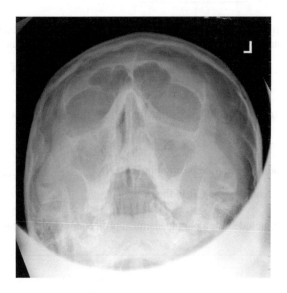

107. Figure 11-28: _____

_____

_____

_____

Figure 11-29

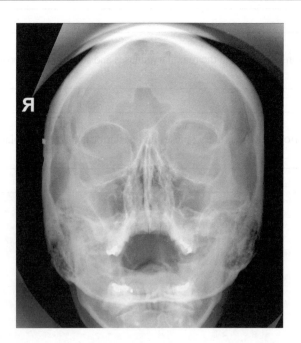

108. Figure 11-29, parietocanthial: _____

_____

_____

_____

Figure 11-30

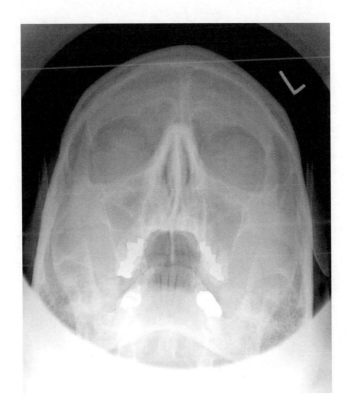

109. Figure 11-30, parietocanthial: _____

_____

_____